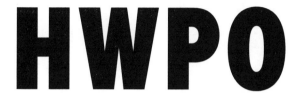

HARD WORK PAYS OFF

MAT FRASER

with Spenser Mestel
Recipes by Sammy Moniz
Illustrations by David Regone

RODALE
New York

Library of Congress Cataloging-in-Publication Data has been applied for.

ISBN 978-0-593-23375-7
Ebook ISBN 978-0-593-23376-4

Printed in the United States of America

Book design by Andrea Lau
Illustrations by David Regone
Cover design by Pete Garceau
Cover photograph courtesy of Rogue Fitness

10 9 8 7 6 5 4 3 2

First Edition

To Sammy, for loving me regardless of what place I got.

CONTENTS

CrossFit Games Champion Personal Records

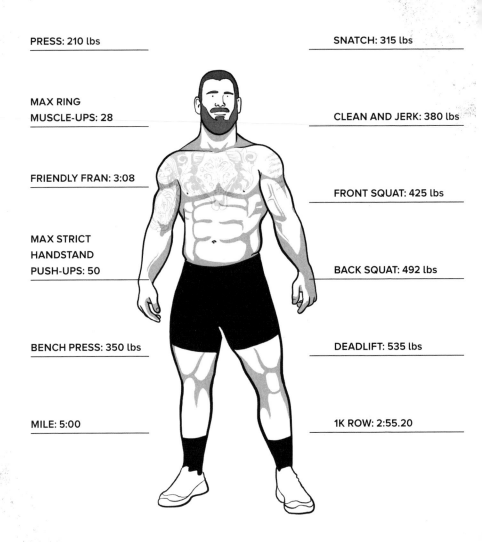

PRESS: 210 lbs

SNATCH: 315 lbs

MAX RING
MUSCLE-UPS: 28

CLEAN AND JERK: 380 lbs

FRIENDLY FRAN: 3:08

FRONT SQUAT: 425 lbs

MAX STRICT
HANDSTAND
PUSH-UPS: 50

BACK SQUAT: 492 lbs

BENCH PRESS: 350 lbs

DEADLIFT: 535 lbs

MILE: 5:00

1K ROW: 2:55.20

3: Speed

4: Coordination

Introduction

The decision to keep competing after the 2015 season seems so obvious now, but that's not how I felt at the end of that year's CrossFit Games.

After the last event, while I was still gasping for air, I lay down on a supply cart in the athlete tunnel and replayed in my head all the mistakes I'd made. A few had been purely physical. I couldn't sprint. I could barely swim. Of all the guys on the field, I had one of the weakest deadlifts.

But the worst ones had been mental. When we had to flip the 560-pound "Pig" down the soccer field for the eighth event, I couldn't figure out the right technique, so I panicked. I did most of the work with my biceps, gassed myself out, and gave up a huge part of my lead. Then I got rattled again on the last event. After I failed one handstand push-up after another, I never thought to take a break, recover, and readjust the parallettes. So I kept failing, and even going full dummy on the Assault Bike and rower wasn't enough. For the second year in a row, I came in second.

I was disappointed, humiliated, and ready to quit. I knew that

I'd lost—or maybe it's more accurate to say that I'd choked—because I'd cut corners, and if I wanted to make another run at the Games, I'd have to be all in. Obviously, that meant more training in my tiny home gym, by myself, with no one around to slap me on the ass and tell me "good job." I'd also have to stop thinking I was the expert and seek out new coaches to help me attack my weaknesses, which was why the first step to a comeback would be so brutal. I'd have to do what I did after every competition: watch the footage and create a list of everything that I'd done wrong. Did I really want to become a champion that badly?

I mean, this wasn't the first dream that hadn't panned out for me. After a decade of weightlifting and years at the Olympic Training Center, I didn't make the Olympic team, and that didn't kill me, right? Plus, I had two university degrees, and even though I'd hated my summer internship at an aerospace company, I was sure I could find an engineering job I liked. Or I could even go back to working in the oil fields in Alberta.

I didn't have to kill myself in the gym every day. I didn't have to keep doing rowing intervals that were so intense I left literal puddles of sweat on the floor. I didn't have to restructure my life around one singular goal: to win the CrossFit Games.

I wanted a normal life. I wanted to go to my friend's bachelor party without worrying about missing training, drive to Rhode Island to see my girlfriend whenever I felt like it, and spend my rest days waterskiing, not on top of a lacrosse ball for twelve hours rolling out the tension in my muscles.

I'm sure these excuses sound familiar. They're what you tell yourself when you're too tired to make the 7 a.m. class or too hungover to even consider a Sunday-morning lifting session. They're the excuses everyone makes, and I made them all throughout the 2015 season.

But then I changed. Lying on that supply cart after the last event, choking back tears as the other competitors streamed past, I knew I never again wanted to feel as low as I did in that moment. To avoid that possibility completely, I had two options: I could quit CrossFit altogether and start looking for a desk job.

Or I could radically transform my mindset. Every choice I was faced with, I would ask myself whether it would help me win the CrossFit Games. No? Then I wouldn't do it.

And now, after eight years in the sport, I'm the most successful competitive CrossFit athlete in history. I've won more events (29), more titles (5 in a row), and by the largest margins of anyone in the sport.

While there are some guys who might beat me in a single workout, no one can say they're a better all-around athlete. Weightlifting, gymnastics, kettlebells, running, swimming, rowing, strongman: I've relentlessly trained them all, so now you don't have to guess how to.

While competing, I would never have offered this information and risked giving the other athletes an edge. But now that I've decided to retire from professional CrossFit, I can finally share with you how I prepared my body and trained my mind.

Needless to say, it won't be easy. After the 2015 Games, I bought my own Pig and flipped it every night after everyone had gone home. The impact from catching the 560-pound mat was so intense on my hands that I went to the doctor and got X-rays. He thought I'd punched a wall with both fists.

Except for a few weeks I'd take off in August, every day for the past five years was roughly the same: wake up earlier than I'd like, sell my soul to the Assault Bike and the swimming intervals and the 40-minute AMRAPs, eat, sleep, repeat.

But it absolutely was worth it. CrossFit is how I met my best friends, business partners, and even my wife. CrossFit is how I found the artist who tattooed my chest, how I was able to travel across the world, and how I bought our home. CrossFit is also one of the most supportive communities I've ever been a part of.

During the Games, when I was on the competition floor trying to hold on to the barbell for the last few reps of the workout and so overheated that my head felt like it was being crushed in a vise, it was the fans who helped me get across the finish line.

So what I'm telling you is something you've already heard but may not fully understand: Hard work pays off.

How to Use This Guide

Take This Book to the Gym

This book is meant to be your total training manual, so take it to the gym. Write your PRs (personal records) in the margins. Circle the techniques you need to master. And most of all, do the workouts. They come from my last five years of preparing for and winning the CrossFit Games, and if the workouts at the end of each section aren't enough, there's an appendix in the back with even more (along with a glossary for any terms that might be unfamiliar). The deadlift technique work, the swimming kick intervals, the high-knee drills, the scap push-ups—all of them helped me become a champion.

You'll also see prompts for journal entries throughout the book. When there's a problem I need to solve, I write until I've figured it out, and I encourage you to do the same.

Infinitely Scalable

One of the best parts of CrossFit is that it's "infinitely scalable," meaning pretty much anyone—from a newbie to a Games athlete—can do the same workout. Take "Fran," one of our most infamous workouts. I do it "Rx" (i.e., the way it was originally written), and that means 21 thrusters at 95 pounds and 21 pull-ups, then 15 thrusters and 15 pull-ups, and finally 9 thrusters and 9 pull-ups.

But this is meant to be an all-out sprint—I do it in about two minutes—so if you know that 45 total thrusters would take you, say, 12 minutes, you should drop the weight. And if you've never done more than a few pull-ups before, you'd probably use an elastic band for a little bit of assistance. And if this is your first time ever doing CrossFit, and you're asking yourself, "What the hell is a thruster?" don't worry. You'll be doing air squats and jumping pull-ups.

So even though I'm presently the best in the world at CrossFit and can probably hit this workout heavier and faster than you, we can all do it side by side—the Games athlete, the weekend warrior, the average CrossFit athlete, and the newbie. Our weights and movements may seem different, but we're all trying to improve in the same ways: quicker transitions, more efficient technique, better breathing patterns.

Making Progress

No matter how fit you are, you can still become fitter, and that's how this book is structured. Each section starts with the fundamentals, which you may be eager to skip. Don't. I've intentionally left out "elite" scaling options here because even the best athletes should build a solid foundation before they move on.

As each section progresses, the scaling options start to fall off. This also isn't an accident. I'm trying to prevent you from making the same mistakes I did by forcing you to build the strength, stamina, and technique necessary to scale up. For example, if you've never done a parallette handstand push-up, you must practice a strict handstand push-up first.

When it comes to the weight you should use, many of the workouts include a percentage that's based on your one-rep max, the most you can lift for a certain movement. This number will probably change (hopefully by going up), so you'll want to retest it every few months and adjust your weight accordingly.

Other workouts are considered CrossFit benchmarks, which are meant to be done periodically to see how and where you're improving. They have prescribed "men's" and "women's" weights, along with a scaling option, so I'm going to give you those numbers as a reference. But they may not be appropriate for you, so I'm also going to include my best time for the workout to give you a general sense of how long it should take you. Then you can scale accordingly.

You may also see workouts with movements you haven't learned yet, like in "Mary," which has handstand push-ups, one-legged squats (pistols), and pull-ups. Scale them by looking at what came earlier in the chapter, like ring rows before pull-ups.

Learning how to modify a workout is its own skill, so you may struggle with it at first. That's okay. You can always practice more with the workouts in the appendix. They don't have weights, just general guidelines like "light" or "medium-heavy," so they're a great way to experiment with different loads.

Throughout the book, I've also embedded some of my personal stories and the lessons I've learned. Hopefully some of them will resonate with you.

1

Strength

For my first five years of weightlifting, every part of my training was focused on technique. My starting position, my pull from the ground, my bar path as it traveled up—everything had to be perfect, and I hated it. I started weightlifting because I wanted to get jacked, not to have the best form. But now, almost a decade after I quit that sport, I see how much that foundation paid off.

Just by looking at a workout, I know exactly how to adjust my technique. If the weight is light and the reps are high, I can shorten my movement and cycle the bar as quickly as possible. If the weight is heavy or I need to recover, I can switch to slow, efficient single reps. And whether I'm fresh or at the end of a workout, I never need to worry about not meeting the movement standards—the infamous "no rep."

However, technique alone wasn't enough to make me great. When I went to the Olympic Training Camp, I was the weakest guy by far, which is how I ended up breaking my back in two places. From then all the way through my CrossFit career, I've had to dedicate myself to strength—sometimes to the exclusion of all else. It's a long, repetitive process, but to be your best self, you need both strength and technique.

I'm here to teach you both.

Strength Technique 101

WORKOUT: *The Clean Starting Position*

15 Reps
Pull a PVC pipe from the ground to the hang

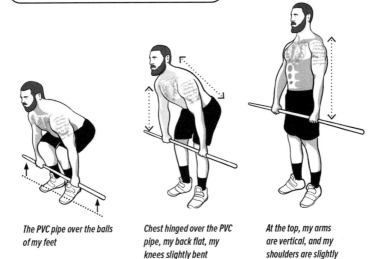

The PVC pipe over the balls of my feet

Chest hinged over the PVC pipe, my back flat, my knees slightly bent

At the top, my arms are vertical, and my shoulders are slightly in front of the bar

My weightlifting career began by accident. In middle school, my best friend and I were on the football team, and for a few days each week, we'd get to lift with the high school guys. There was

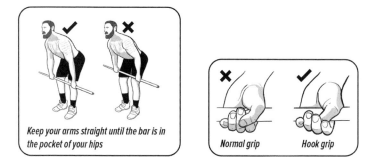

Keep your arms straight until the bar is in the pocket of your hips

Normal grip   Hook grip

no training program to follow, so each session we'd max out our bench press and do bicep curls until we failed. At that age, your body's growing so quickly that you don't need good form to get stronger. Almost every time I lifted, I'd hit a new personal record.

During one of these sessions, a football coach saw my passion and suggested to my dad, who along with my mom was a former Olympic athlete, that I train at an actual weightlifting club. At the time, I had no clue how any of the movements were supposed to look, and I didn't even know I was already doing a "clean and jerk." I just thought it was cool to get the barbell from the ground over my head.

When my dad and I walked into that weightlifting club in Essex, Vermont, it was nothing like what I'd expected. For starters, no one looked like the guys I had seen getting pumped at Muscle Beach. They weren't absolutely shredded, and a lot of them weren't even lifting weights. Instead, they had a PVC pipe in their hands and would do nothing more than bend forward at the waist and stand. Bend at the waist and stand. I didn't even see a rack of dumbbells, just a narrow room with white walls, drop ceilings, and twelve platforms made of unfinished plywood.

I expected I'd train like we did at football practice—no supervision, no form, just lifting as much as I could and dropping the bar when it was too much. Instead, Coach Polakowski told me to grab a broomstick.

For the next few weeks, all I worked on was the starting positions, which differ slightly depending on which of the two Olympic lifts you're doing: the snatch, where you get the barbell from the ground over your head in one motion, or the clean and jerk, where the bar goes first from the ground to your shoulders and then overhead.

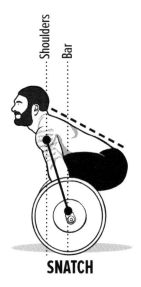

SNATCH

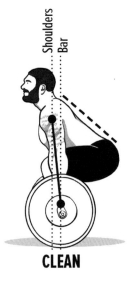

CLEAN

Advanced Technique

EXERCISE
1. The Shrug
2. The High Pull
3. The Muscle Snatch
4. The Power Snatch
5. The Squat

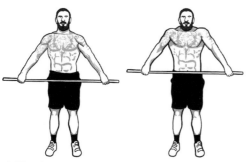

1. The Shrug

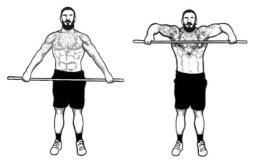

2. The High Pull

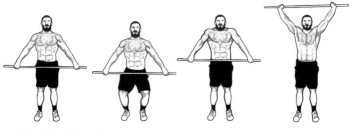

3. The Muscle Snatch

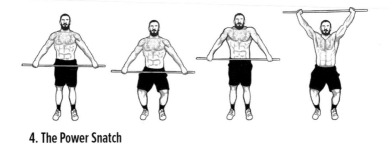

4. The Power Snatch

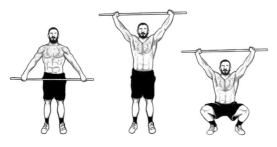

5. The Squat Snatch

I worked on my starting position for weeks, then Coach Pol let me move on to the next step, pulling the stick from the ground to my knees. It was slow, repetitive work, and I hated it. I just kept wondering, "How am I going to get stronger on a broomstick?"

The only encouraging sign was that when Polakowski pointed out where I was making a mistake, I could usually feel it and make a correction. As I'd realize later when I studied engineering in college, my brain is pretty well wired to understand movement. So once Coach Pol gave me the cues, they intuitively made sense.

This body awareness is one of the greatest assets you can have in weightlifting, but I just wanted to set a new PR at every session, especially when I realized how strong the other lifters actually were. Thank goodness Coach Pol prevented me from picking up bad habits that are nearly impossible to break later, like lifting the shoulders too soon or pulling with the arms before the legs are fully extended.

Over the course of months, I graduated from the broomstick to the PVC pipe to the 5- and 7-pound bars, then to the 35-pound bar. At the time, they didn't make bumper plates that were light enough, so I had to use Polakowski's special set, which was homemade and cut out of unpainted plywood. Because the hole for the bar wasn't a perfect circle, the weights would droop to one side like a tree blown over by the wind.

Thankfully, companies like Rogue now sell training bars and bumper plates meant for kids who are even younger than I was when I started, so you don't have to make your own. But if you're going to let your preteen snatch and clean and jerk, make sure they've got plenty of supervision. If not, they may end up with the type of injury that almost ended my athletic career.

EXERCISE: *Power Snatch*

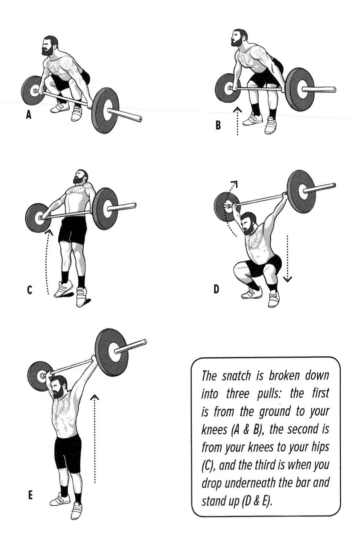

The snatch is broken down into three pulls: the first is from the ground to your knees (A & B), the second is from your knees to your hips (C), and the third is when you drop underneath the bar and stand up (D & E).

EXERCISE: *Hang Power Snatch*

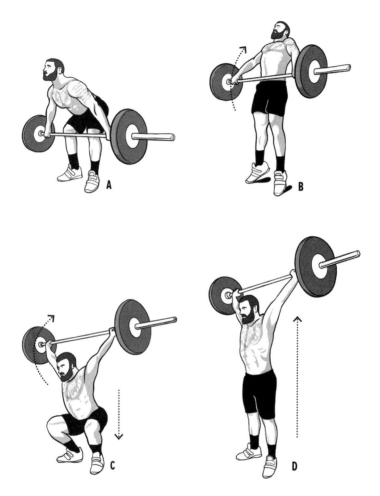

Around the same time as I was weightlifting, I was also playing football. Even though I wasn't the tallest guy, I could pack muscle onto my frame and still sprint pretty quickly, but there was a huge obstacle I never overcame: my compromised hearing.

All the other kids had played football or grew up watching it, so they understood the rhythm. I didn't. Plus, in the huddle I almost never heard which play we were going to run. Sometimes I was able to ask the quarterback before he snapped the ball, but usually I had no idea what was about to happen. By the time I got to high school, the coaches just told me to line up wherever I wanted on the defensive line and then overpower the other guys. I did, but it's hard to feel like a part of the team when you know there's something you're missing.

Thankfully, this was never an issue with Coach Pol. If you missed a lift at a meet, he'd take the time to explain why, and I became one of the country's best lifters in my weight class.

Since it was clear I had a future in the sport, my next decision was easy. There's only one place to go with Olympic weightlifting, and it's to the Olympics, so I applied for Team USA's Olympic Training Center in Colorado Springs.

In 2008, the day I graduated from high school, my dad and I drove west. I was eighteen and the youngest lifter invited to train with Team USA, which was about to compete in the Beijing Games. Sponsorship money was pouring into the OTC, and I was shocked the first time I walked into the training room and they told me I could take a Gatorade. *Like, for free?* I asked. *Yeah,* they said. *Take two.* I grabbed a whole case, and a few weeks later, I nabbed something else.

In addition to my partial deafness, I was also born with terrible eyesight. I didn't realize it at first. I just thought that you weren't supposed to see the leaves on trees or what was written on the blackboard in class if you were sitting farther away than the first row. I'd always get in trouble for looking at the paper of the kid next to me, but I truly had no idea what the teacher was writing. Eventually, though, I got glasses, and when I found out that contacts were free at the OTC, I took them by the box. I wore them as long as possible—even when I would swim without goggles—and they ended up lasting me six years.

EXERCISE: *Snatch Balance*

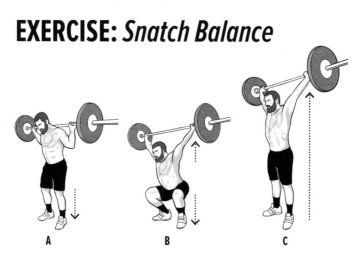

A **B** **C**

The Snatch Balance is a great drill to improve your third pull. To do it, rack the barbell on your traps behind your head with your feet at shoulder-width (A). Then, while keeping your torso upright, bend your knees like you're doing a push press. As you jump your feet into a squat stance, drop underneath the barbell as quickly as possible and lock your elbow so the bar ends up above your head (B). Stabilize the barbell if you need to and then stand up (C).

Though the perks were great, the volume of training was more than I'd expected. To warm up, we did a ton of jumping to activate our fast-twitch muscles, then we'd do about 24 snatches. For me, that meant 2 sets of 3 at 115 pounds, 2 sets of 3 at 135 pounds, doubles at 155, 185, 205, and 225, then a couple of singles after that. Every third session, we'd practice our clean and jerk, and the rep scheme would be essentially the same.

This is similar to what I'd done in Vermont, but we were now

WORKOUT: *SNATCH COMPLEX*

Every *1: 15* **for 7 sets**
1 Power Snatch @77%
1 Hang Power Snatch @77%
2 Snatch Balance @77%

Power Snatch

Hang Power Snatch

Snatch Balance

doing all this twice a day. If you factored in the accessory work and body maintenance, training could easily be six hours a day, six days a week.

WORKOUT: *Power Snatch*

1 × 3 @ 80%
2 × 3 @ 85%
1 × 2 @ 80%
3 × 2 @ 75 %

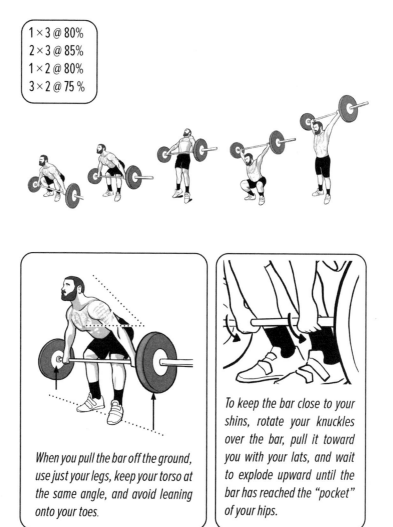

When you pull the bar off the ground, use just your legs, keep your torso at the same angle, and avoid leaning onto your toes.

To keep the bar close to your shins, rotate your knuckles over the bar, pull it toward you with your lats, and wait to explode upward until the bar has reached the "pocket" of your hips.

The goal of all the training volume was to make the movements feel automatic. That takes years to learn. Including the lifts from my CrossFit career, I've done probably 60,000 snatches in my life and half as many clean and jerks, which had a huge payoff. When I approach the bar, I'm not conscious of any specific cues. I'm not thinking about rotating my knuckles over the bar or exploding upward on my second pull. If I clear my mind completely, I know my form will be tight. That's how comfortable you want to be with the lift.

To make sure your technique is always uniform, I recommend developing a pre-lift routine. To start, I put my left foot under the bar before my right. Then I grab the bar with my right hand before the left. Some athletes like to take a static start, where they're completely still before they initiate the lift. I like to do it dynamically, and as I hinge at the waist, I bend and straighten my legs—quick hip pumps that help me feel the stretch in my muscles. Then I count down in my head: 3, 2, 1, go. Ideally, everything is on autopilot from then on.

After eight months at the OTC, I was told I'd have to hit two PRs and qualify for the Junior World Team if I wanted to stay in Colorado Springs. The numbers they wanted me to hit were so much higher than where I was at, and building that kind of strength takes time.

That's why I'm so surprised by how some CrossFit athletes train. They hit 90 to 95 percent of their max every session. That's not how you get better. Especially for the Olympic lifts, the sweet spot is in the 70 to 80 percent range, maybe a little heavier for snatches, but not usually above 85 percent.

WORKOUT: *Back Squat*

6×2 @ 80%

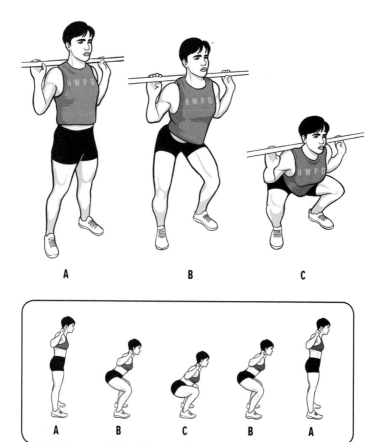

A B C

A B C B A

You also need to build your foundation for strength. When I first got to the OTC, my clean and jerk PR was about 150 kilos, or 330 pounds, and my deadlift was right around that. Deadlift is typically your heaviest lift by a lot, but we never trained it as part of our programming, not even at the OTC. So before the qualifications for Junior Worlds, I spent more time than ever doing that kind of pure strength work, which was a huge stress on my central nervous system.

I ended up qualifying for the Junior World Team, but about a month before we left, I was doing heavy clean pulls at 376 pounds. These were essentially my one-rep max deadlift, but at the top of the lift I'd also have to explode upward onto my toes to get the barbell as high as possible.

The strain on my back was too much, and I heard a loud pop on my left side. I'd just broken the left "wing" of my L-5, but I wouldn't realize that for a few more months. At the time, all I knew was that something was seriously wrong, but my coach told me it was too late to sub in an alternate, so I sucked down Motrin like they were Pez and kept lifting.

Then, right before we flew out, I was in the bottom of a heavy squat when I heard a second pop. I'd just broken the right wing.

I still competed in Romania—but not well. In addition to my broken back, I also had strep throat, and I was barely able to hit my opening weights. It was a disaster of a meet, and in retrospect I was lucky that it wasn't even worse. When I eventually found a spinal surgeon to repair the break, Dr. Bray told me that my L-5 could've slipped forward and out of alignment at any time. If that had happened, they would've had to fuse it to the vertebra above it, limiting the range of motion in my back and probably ending my athletic career.

WORKOUT: *Clean and Jerk*

5 rounds
1 Squat Clean + 2 Split Jerks
3 @ 77%
1 @ 80%
1 @ 75%

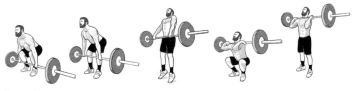

Squat Clean

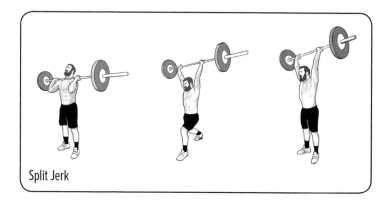

Split Jerk

As it was, all the spinal surgeons I saw around the OTC—in Denver, Boulder, and Colorado Springs—wanted me to get that fusion. One said that I was done lifting and would be lucky to jog again without pain. By pure coincidence, though, Dr. Bray was visiting the OTC right as I was about to leave for winter break and told me about an experimental surgery.

Because he had to do it while the bones were still growing, it was practically guaranteed to work on a seventeen-year-old and guaranteed to fail on a twenty-three-year-old. I was right in the middle so I had about a fifty-fifty chance. I booked the surgery for a few weeks later. Two days before Christmas, he drilled into my spine and installed a tiny plate using a procedure that was so precise that it barely left a scar. Still, recovery was long and slow, but I learned two important lessons.

The first is that gritting through pain is an unavoidable part of any sport, but there's a point at which you have to listen to your body and slow down or stop altogether. If my mom hadn't eventually intervened and demanded that I get a full X-ray on my back, who knows how long I would've trained with it before seeing Dr. Bray.

Second, no one is ever going to take your goals as seriously as you. I'm sure the other spinal surgeons were doing what they thought was best, but at the end of the day, it wasn't their back that they were going to operate on. Regardless of whether it's your coach, teammates, or doctor, remember that the ultimate responsibility for your health falls on you, not them.

WORKOUT: *Fran*

21–15–9
Thrusters (M 95 lbs/W 65 lbs)
Pull-Ups
My time: about *3:00*

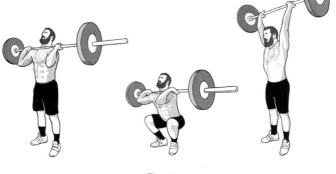

Thrusters

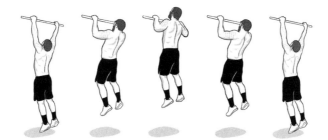

Pull-Ups

EXERCISE: *Thruster*

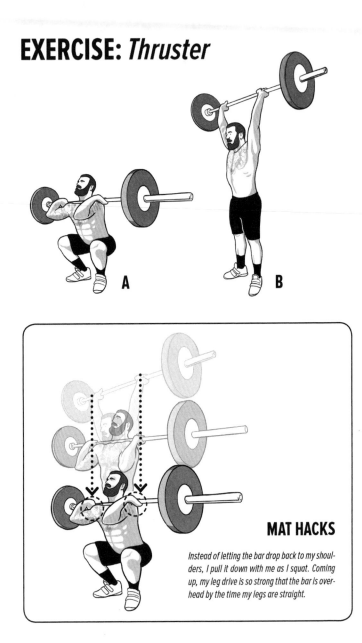

A

B

MAT HACKS

Instead of letting the bar drop back to my shoulders, I pull it down with me as I squat. Coming up, my leg drive is so strong that the bar is overhead by the time my legs are straight.

Thankfully, I fully recovered from my back surgery and was able to transfer to the Olympic Education Center at Northern Michigan University, in the Upper Peninsula. Even before the injury, I knew that I wanted to get a college or university degree, which wasn't possible taking one class a semester at the OTC. Academics were a bigger priority at Marquette, and the coach was willing to give me a spot on the team while I rehabbed my back. So that's where I spent the next two years.

Arriving at NMU, I knew in the back of my mind that making the Olympic team was unlikely. Especially after the surgery, I just wasn't strong enough and didn't have adequate time to train before qualifications. Still, I kept lifting, mostly because it was all that I knew. Plus, I was getting an education, at least until 2011, when Team USA announced that our funding was getting cut. That's when I decided to transfer to the University of Vermont, where I'd get free tuition because my mom was a member of the faculty. But so few of my credits transferred that, even though I'd been taking classes for the past three years, I was basically a sophomore. That was a tough blow.

Not only was I moving back in with my parents after failing to make the Olympics, but also all my old friends were either working or just finishing college. I felt like I was years behind. After a lifetime of sports, I was also sitting on my butt more than I ever had before. So I found a nearby gym, Champlain Valley CrossFit. The owner, Jade Jenny, was willing to let me do my Olympic lifts off to the side. I wasn't interested in CrossFit, so I tried to be there in the off-hours when I wouldn't be in the way.

WORKOUT: *Heavy Grace*

As Fast as Possible
30 Clean and Jerks (M 225 lbs/W 155 lbs)
My time: *1:18*

The goal for normal "Grace" is to use a weight that allows you to finish in four to eight minutes, faster if you're a Games athlete. For "Heavy Grace," you want to add between 33% and 66% more to the bar.

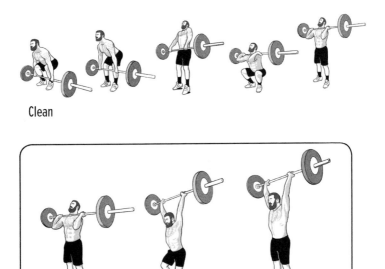

Clean

Jerk

One day, though, I couldn't avoid it, and what I saw shook me. Weightlifting is a very controlled sport. If someone's about to attempt a heavy lift, no one moves or speaks. But that day in the gym, the class appeared to be pure chaos. The music was just as loud as the weights crashing to the ground, and everyone was hopping over one another's barbells as they ran to do their pull-ups.

This was actually the perfect introduction, the mindset you need for CrossFit. If you want to be competitive, you've got to learn how to filter out the mayhem, even when a dozen other athletes are on the floor beside you. That was one of the biggest shifts I had to make between the OTC and CrossFit. The other was learning how to breathe.

Weight lifters never do cardio. In fact, we're encouraged to sit for minutes between our sets, so I really underestimated how much I'd suffer when a guy from the gym suggested we do "Grace." He told me it was the "heavy" version, but I wasn't nervous. I could do a 225-pound clean and jerk when I was thirteen years old, so I loaded the bar and expected to do one right after the other. How long could that take? Ninety seconds?

Not only did this workout humble me, but I also learned perhaps the most important lesson when it comes to strength in CrossFit: It means next to nothing when your heart rate spikes to 200 beats per minute. As anyone who's ever done Grace will know, I didn't do one rep right after the other. By the time I was six minutes in, I'd never felt pain like that in my lungs, and I failed one of the last clean and jerks, something I hadn't done since I was a teenager. I was wrecked but also hungry. Something I thought would be easy that ended up kicking me in the face? I gotta try that again.

At this point, I was starting to come around on CrossFit. From doing just a few classes a week, I was seeing improvement, even if it was just a little bit, and I was also starting to win some local competitions. That was huge for me. Though it wasn't a lot of prize money, I was the definition of a broke college kid. I drove a used car, didn't have a job, and had to ask my parents for money every time I wanted to go out to eat.

Plus, there was no money in Olympic lifting. Guys would travel here from Russia to try to earn $5,000 at the Arnold Sports Festival in Columbus, so when Jade told me that I could win $500 at Champlain Valley's Winter Throwdown, I was ready to throw down. But I didn't even have the $50 entry fee.

Jade told me he'd waive it if I promised to buy real CrossFit shoes if I won. I did, I bought the shoes, and from then on I was looking for every competition I could. There were times when I'd fly out as far as Minnesota on Friday morning, take a red-eye back on Sunday night, and go straight from the airport to my first class at UVM. It was an exhausting lifestyle, but I couldn't believe I could make pocket money by working out. In fact, I'm still so grateful I had the opportunity to earn a living doing what I loved, and it all started that year with my first CrossFit Open.

That year, Jade knew me well enough to guess that I wouldn't sign up on my own. At the time, I didn't even know what it was, let alone realize that it's the largest fitness competition in the world, with practically every one of the roughly 15,000 affiliates in the world doing the workouts as they're announced each week.

Thankfully, Jade saw that I had potential and signed up for me. He knew he'd have to hold my hand the entire way, including counting my reps and screaming at me to stop resting, but I

WORKOUT: *13.1*

AMRAP in *17:00*
40 Burpees
30 Snatches (M 75 lbs/W 45 lbs)
30 Burpees
30 Snatches (M 135 lbs/W /75 lbs)
20 Burpees
30 Snatches (M 165 lbs/W 100 lbs)
10 Burpees
Max Snatches (M 210 lbs/W 120 lbs)
My time: time-capped, with 3 Burpees left

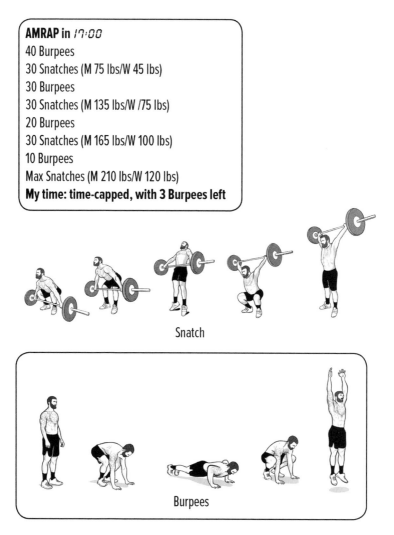

Snatch

Burpees

didn't appreciate that dedication at the time. Instead, I blew off the workouts he programmed for me and did whatever I wanted in the lead-up to the Open. Thankfully, he stuck with me.

Since that season, 2013, the structure for competitive CrossFit has changed pretty much every year, but the basics have stayed the same. If you do well in the Open, you move on. Now it's the top 10 percent who qualify for the next round, but before 2021, you had to be in the .01 percent. In 2013, that meant 40 men and women from each region would go to the next competition (out of about 100,000 athletes total), then 3 of them would make it to the Games.

Again, I didn't know any of that when Jade told me I'd be doing an Open workout every Friday for the next five weeks. I also didn't realize that these workouts are especially grueling, but I'd learn that quickly, along with relearning the lesson about humility from when I did "Heavy Grace."

On paper, the first workout, 13.1, looked like a cakewalk: snatches that got progressively heavier but topped off at 210, about 90 pounds lighter than my one-rep max. So I was half listening when Jade told me how to break up the workout. *Yeah, right,* I thought. *I'm going to smash these burpees and rep out as many snatches at 210 as possible.* If I could manage that, Jade told me, I could probably set the world record.

The workout started with 40 burpees, more than I'd ever done in a row before, and that's when I knew I was in trouble. I couldn't get my breath under control, not even when I moved on to the lightest snatches, and after I finished the set at 165, I had only a minute left to do 10 burpees.

When I compete today, I do a burpee in three seconds, two if it's the end of the workout and I can drop the hammer without having to worry about recovering. But that day, no. It hurt too badly, and once I was on the floor, no amount of screaming from Jade was going to get me back up again. It took me the full 60 seconds to do seven burpees, no time to attempt even one snatch at 210.

This is another part of CrossFit that a lot of athletes seem to forget: A one-rep max is a lot of fun, but you're almost never going to do it during a workout. Yeah, there are a few exceptions now and then, but even at the Games, it's more likely to be a speed ladder, where you have to hit one lift right after the other. So if you want to be successful in this sport, don't train like you're at the OTC. Make sure you can hit your biggest lifts under fatigue.

CrossFit Games Strength

Through the 2013 Open, I beat out thousands of other athletes and qualified for Regionals, the last stage before the CrossFit Games. They were in Boston that year, and again Jade was my coach. Knowing that I still had zero aerobic capacity, he told me to hold a conservative pace on the row of the first event, Jackie. I did, which left me sitting and staring as pretty much every other guy got off the rower, grabbed the barbell and started doing his thrusters. I hated being last, but I hoped that I could cycle the barbell better than anyone else.

For maybe the first time in my CrossFit career up until that point, my expectations were right. Even though 45 pounds was light weight for everyone on the floor that day, I moved twice as quickly. Instead of letting the bar drop back to my shoulders after the press-out at the top, I pulled it down with me as I squatted. Coming up, my leg drive was so strong that the bar was overhead by the time my legs were straight. Any deficit I had from the row, I more than made up for on the thrusters, which hammered home for me the importance of proper barbell cycling.

There's a surprising number of techniques you can use to do the barbell lifts. For example, the fastest way to finish Isabel (30 snatches) is one snatch after another ("unbroken") without bending your knees and dropping underneath the barbell. This variation is called a "muscle snatch" because you have to pull the bar all the way above your head using your shoulders. To go even faster, don't even bring the barbell all the way to your hips (definitely not what Coach Pol taught me). Instead, touch it only to

WORKOUT: *Jackie*

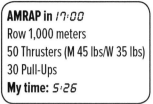

AMRAP in *17:00*
Row 1,000 meters
50 Thrusters (M 45 lbs/W 35 lbs)
30 Pull-Ups
My time: *5:26*

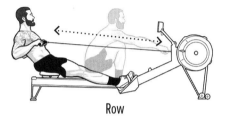

Row

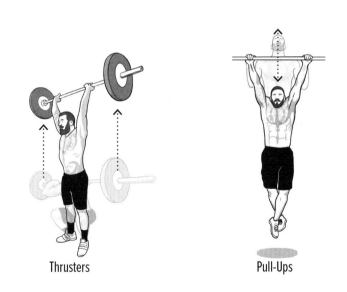

Thrusters   Pull-Ups

your thighs on the way up and down. This is feasible only if the weight is extremely light for you—think 45 percent of your one-rep max.

WORKOUT: *Isabel*

> **AMRAP**
> 30 Snatches (M 135 lbs/W 95 lbs)

A

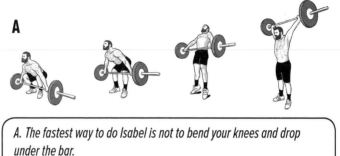

> A. The fastest way to do Isabel is not to bend your knees and drop under the bar.

B

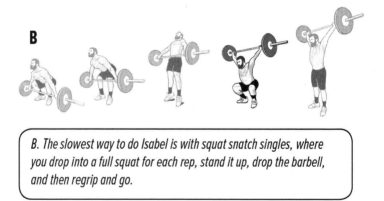

> B. The slowest way to do Isabel is with squat snatch singles, where you drop into a full squat for each rep, stand it up, drop the barbell, and then regrip and go.

Because there's so much more movement involved, this is exhausting from an aerobic point of view but allows you to keep hitting a heavy weight.

In between these two options, there's a lot of variability. You can power snatch sets of 5. You can muscle snatch with a hip touch for 15 reps and then go to singles. The only way to know the best method is to experiment with all of them, so adjust the weights for Isabel and see what works. Then when snatches come up in a workout, you'll have a full set of options. Just remember: You're trying to optimize both speed and energy input, so what's quickest isn't necessarily the best in every circumstance.

Learning how to cycle the barbell efficiently and consistently is so important that I program my training around it. As I get deeper into a workout, I'll give myself either more rest or shorter sets, but I have to speed up my cycle time each round. Doing this gives me the confidence to know that, even if I'm at the tail end of a 30-minute workout, I'm not conditioned to feel the fatigue and put my hands on my knees or go chalk my hands. I may be catching a snatch lower because I have less hip drive, but the technique—and the barbell cycling—is exactly the same.

Remember, cycling isn't just for barbells. At the 2019 Games, I knew the second event was going to be fast. When it's only 800 meters, all the top guys can row at a similar pace, and most can finish that handstand walk without a lot of difficulties, so I was pretty sure that the workout would be won or lost at the kettlebell jerks. Because sixty-six reps is a lot, even a half second on each rep was going to be decisive.

Instead of pausing at the top of the jerk to show that I'd

completed the rep, I decided to go as quickly as possible. So while everyone around me was driving from their knees and keeping their torsos perfectly upright, like you generally should for a jerk, I leaned my torso back and forth and essentially strict-pressed the kettlebells. It was risky—I got no-repped a decent number of times—but still quicker overall than the full range of motion would've been.

Still, barbell cycling can take you only so far. If you're looking to become an elite competitor, you'll probably have to take time off from your other training to focus exclusively on strength. That's what I did after the 2016 Games when I reached out to powerlifting legend Chad Wesley Smith, owner and founder of Juggernaut Training Systems, and asked him for help with my deadlift.

In terms of technique, Smith could already guess what my problem was going to be. He's coached more than two hundred seminars and seen a ton of CrossFit athletes, so he knows that the first pull of our deadlift almost always looks like the start of a clean. Those two lifts may seem similar, but in the deadlift, you're hinged more at the hips, so you have a higher hip position. In a clean, your hips are lower and your chest should be higher.

The good news was that the muscles I needed to deadlift were already strong. I just had to teach them how to move in the right ways. Because I knew I'd be more likely to do large sets at an intermediate weight, as opposed to a one-rep max, we focused on the former by doing max reps off a six-inch block, which made the lift easier. The next week, the barbell went to a four-inch block, then two inches, then the floor. Each time, I had to hit the same number of reps, and I did this program for five months.

The results were huge. Not only did I have a higher one-rep max and greater capacity to crank out deadlifts, but my core was also much stronger, which had huge payoffs. Before, if I got stuck at the bottom of a clean, I just did squats, squats, squats. But my legs weren't the weakness; my core was, and all my lifts—front squat, back squat, snatch—felt easier after training with Smith. If you want to strengthen your own core, check out the ab exercises at the end of this section.

WORKOUT: *Power Ladder*

1-rep Max Clean

Adrenaline is one hell of a drug. When a one-rep clean was announced as the eighth event of the 2019 Games, I wasn't feeling overly confident. Not only was I in second place overall, but also the guy in first, Noah Ohlsen, had just come off three big finishes, and I knew the following morning we'd be swimming, a strength of his. I had to make a strong showing and stop the bleeding, but during the season, the heaviest I'd cleaned was about 345, which wouldn't get me past the fourth round of this ladder.

I hit the first four weights, which is when I expected most of the other guys to start dropping out. But everyone kept making their lifts—until we got to 365. That's when Noah got pinned in the hole and couldn't stand up the bar. Because he tied with another guy, they went to the tiebreaker: Whoever did five reps at 295 pounds the quickest would take fifth in the event.

WORKOUT: *Deadlifts*

> **Every 3 minutes for 5 sets**
> 5 @ 65%
> 3 @ 75%
> 1 @ 82%

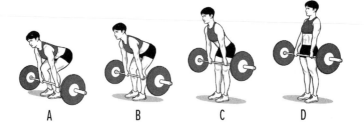

A   B   C   D

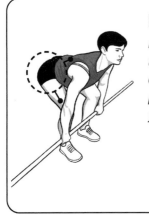

MAT HACKS

In the deadlift, you're hinged more at the hips than you would be for the clean or the snatch. So start with a higher hip position and feel the movement more in your glutes, hamstrings, and lower back.

Ohlsen won by three-hundredths of a second. That didn't give me a lot of points to gain on him even if I won the event, but at least I could start the climb back to first place.

I made 370 and then 375, which left just me and Scott Pan-chik. If we both hit the next weight, I would lose. I'd seen Panchik power clean 335 from a hang, so I knew he'd obliterate me in the tiebreaker. I didn't think that I could do 380, either, but that's my favorite position to be in: back against the fence, nothing to lose.

Scott missed his attempt at 380, and I was so fired up that I felt like I could've snatched the bar if I'd had to. Before they called my name, energy was pouring out of me—adjusting my lifting belt, rubbing my hands, shaking my head, pumping my fists—and then I walked to the platform. This was everything that Olympic lifting meets were not: 1,000 flashes and 10,000 cheers from everyone in the stadium. Still, my routine was the same. Left foot under the bar, then the right. Right hand, left hand, pump the hips and count down from 3, 2, 1. "He hits this, he wins the event," a commentator said as I landed in my squat. And then I stood up.

It's one of my all-time favorite memories of competition, and I never could've gotten there on my own. If we'd been able to choose our own weights, there was no chance I would've said 380. I would've gone 340, 350, maybe 365—and I would've been shocked to stand that up.

So when you feel like you're way out of your league, see that as an opportunity to make a statement, if not to anyone but yourself. Your back's against the wall. You've got nothing to lose.

The Strength Mentality

JOURNAL ENTRY—What are your "bad" motivators, the ones you think you "shouldn't" have, the ones that you're too ashamed to admit out loud?

I didn't start doing CrossFit because I thought I'd become the five-time champion. That would come later. What got me showing up to the gym on that first day was that I was lonely, bored, out of shape, and looking to fall back into some good habits. And the only reason I started competing was that Jade paid my entry fee and made me promise to buy real training shoes if I won. And that's okay.

Sometimes you need less-than-perfect reasons to get you in the door, then you can discover your deeper "why." For example, wanting to make some extra pocket cash when I was twenty-three eventually became my mission to provide financial security for me, Sammy, and our future kids, even after I retired from the sport. Like building your foundation of strength, developing a resilient source of motivation takes time and energy.

So let's start at the very beginning: When I ask why you're reading this book, what's the first thing that comes to mind? Maybe because you've got a high school reunion coming up and want to get fit? Or you want to be able to do more push-ups than your co-worker who always brags about how often they go to the gym? Write it down. Just like you can't improve your snatch if you ignore your horrible technique, you can't improve your mindset if you aren't honest with yourself.

Eating for Strength

Will this get me closer to winning the CrossFit Games? That's a question I asked myself every day from 2016 onward, and when it came to being the one who made the decisions about my nutrition, the answer was no. That's why I'm so grateful that Sammy took on that responsibility, along with grocery shopping and even washing the dishes. Especially at the beginning of my career, I really needed the help.

When I first started CrossFit, I had massive fluctuations in weight, from around 170 at my leanest to a bit over 200 when I was trying to put on as much muscle as possible. Each of these had its benefits. Gymnastics movements are easier when you're lighter, and you can usually lift more when you've got more mass. So if strength is your priority, you need plenty of protein: .7 grams per pound of body weight if you're a recreational CrossFit athlete, and probably closer to 1 gram per pound of body weight if you've got your eyes set on being a competitor.

In my case, it wasn't easy finding a way to eat all the protein I needed, on top of training for seven to eight hours a day and doing my prehab and body work. So the food had to be delicious. Following are some of my favorite recipes of Sammy's. This isn't a full meal plan, but it should give you a sense of what I eat when I'm looking to put on more mass—which is ironic, considering that the only reason I started working out as a kid was to lose weight.

Grilled Onion Crunch Burger

1 pound ground beef

1 teaspoon Worcestershire sauce

1 tablespoon umami seasoning

1 onion, large slices

2 ounces sharp cheddar

2 burger buns

2 teaspoons garlic mayo

1 to 2 teaspoons onion crunch chili oil

Sweet potato fries for serving (optional)

1. In a medium bowl, mix the ground beef with the Worcestershire sauce and umami seasoning.
2. Divide the beef mixture into 4 burger patties and allow to sit for 30 minutes for the flavors to marry.
3. Set the grill to medium-high heat. Grill the onions and the burgers, flipping halfway, until desired doneness, 5 to 10 minutes.
4. In the last 1 to 2 minutes of cooking, top each burger with cheddar and allow it to melt.
5. Toast the burger buns in the last 1 to 2 minutes of the burgers cooking.
6. To assemble the burger, spread the mayo and chili oil over each bun, add a layer of onions, and top with a cheeseburger patty.
7. Serve with a side of sweet potato fries, if desired.

I was a pudgy kid, and one day when we were all playing soccer during recess, I kicked the ball and shanked it down the field. "Get the ball, fat-ass," someone yelled at me, and I cried, and I cried. When I got home from school that day, I decided to make a change. I started exercising—and starving myself. I knew nothing about fitness and even less about nutrition, but I'd heard that you should eat only 30 grams of fat a day. That was it, nothing about your age or gender or physical activity, nothing about calories or saturated versus trans fat. Just 30 grams a day, and from the moment I'd wake up, I had a checklist in my brain of how much fat I had left to eat.

Cozy Pot Roast

3 to 4 pounds beef chuck roast, cubed

1 tablespoon salt, plus more for seasoning

1 tablespoon dried parsley

1 teaspoon dried dill

$^1/_2$ teaspoon garlic powder

$^1/_2$ teaspoon onion powder

$^1/_2$ teaspoon black pepper

1 tablespoon olive oil

3 cups beef broth

1 (12-ounce) can cream of mushroom soup

1 pound baby potatoes, halved

1 yellow onion, quartered

1 pound carrots, sliced

Fresh parsley for garnish

Crusty bread for serving (optional)

1. Season the beef with the salt. In a small bowl, mix together the remaining spices (the parsley, dill, garlic powder, onion powder, and black pepper). Sprinkle the seasoning on the beef.
2. Set the pressure cooker to Sear/Sauté and add the olive oil. When the oil shimmers, add the beef to the pot in two batches to brown on all sides for 3 to 5 minutes.
3. Once all the beef is browned, add the beef broth and set the pressure cooker to HIGH. Pressure cook for 20 minutes. Once complete, quick-release the pressure.

4. To the pot, add the cream of mushroom soup, potatoes, onion, and carrots.
5. Set the pressure cooker to HIGH for 3 minutes. Once complete, quick-release.
6. Taste and adjust the salt as needed. Add fresh parsley and serve with crusty bread for dipping, if desired.

At first I started eating plain chicken breasts, bags of spinach, and cans of tuna in water, then I realized that what had the fewest calories was nothing at all. I'd go so long without eating that I'd get light-headed. When I started fainting, it was mostly around the house, but one day I gave a presentation in class and keeled forward, passed out, and split my chin open. My mom told me this was happening because I had low blood sugar, which I took the wrong way. Instead of eating enough food to be healthy, I popped a few Skittles whenever I'd feel woozy.

Traeger Grills Smoked Brisket

1 (12- to 14-pound) whole brisket, trimmed (see Note)

2 tablespoons salt

2 tablespoons fresh ground pepper

2 tablespoons garlic powder

Traeger BBQ sauce of your choice for serving (optional)

1. Preheat the Traeger Grill to 225°F.
2. Generously season the brisket with the salt, pepper, and garlic powder. Place the brisket directly on the grill grates and close the lid. Smoke until the internal temperature reaches 165°F (roughly 5 to 7 hours).
3. Roll out a large piece of butcher paper (or heavy-duty foil). Place the brisket in the center of the paper, roll up the edge, and fold down to create a leakproof seal. Return the brisket to the smoker, place it seam-side down, and allow the weight of the brisket to keep the fold closed.
4. Continue smoking at 225°F until the internal temperature reaches 204°F (roughly 3 to 5 hours).
5. Remove the brisket from the smoker and place on a large cutting board to rest for 30 to 60 minutes.
6. Cut the brisket against the grain. Serve as is or with your favorite Traeger BBQ sauce, if desired.

Note: If you're working with a smaller brisket, simply decrease the amount of seasoning. The cook times will vary only slightly, but on average it should take 11 to 13 hours to reach the finishing temperature, even if you're working with a 6-pound brisket.

Hard Work Pays Off

I don't think Coach Pol knew how restricted my diet was, but he definitely thought it was ridiculous for us lifters to hold back our weight. His philosophy was that we were still growing, so we should feed ourselves accordingly, and he encouraged me to move up a weight class once I was a junior in high school. But I knew that if I moved from the 169-pound division to 187, I'd plummet in the rankings, and I never wanted to take even a half step backward to go three steps forward.

When I finally decided to bump up a weight class, I did it with my usual all-out obsessiveness. For meals, I'd eat as many racks of ribs as possible, and for a snack, I'd take a muffin from Costco (already about 700 calories), pop it into the microwave, then load it up with butter. Before bed each night, I'd eat a full jar of peanut butter, and I could still feel the fat inside my pores when I woke up in the morning. That meal plan "worked" in the sense that I jumped up two weight classes, but it wasn't healthy or sustainable.

Pistachio-Crusted Lamb

2 racks ButcherBox lamb

Salt

2 tablespoons spicy brown mustard

$1/4$ cup crackers or breadcrumbs (I use an
"everything"-seasoned cracker)

$1/4$ cup lightly salted shelled pistachios

1. Preheat the oven to 450°F.
2. Pat each lamb rack dry with a paper towel. Sprinkle with salt to taste. Brush with the spicy brown mustard.
3. Pulse the crackers and pistachios in a blender. Coat each rack with the crumbs, shake off the excess, and lay the rack on a baking sheet bone-side down.
4. Roast at 450°F for 10 minutes. Reduce the oven temperature to 300°F and roast an additional 15 to 20 minutes until the internal temperature reaches 125°F.
5. Remove the racks from the oven and rest for 10 minutes before slicing. Slice between the bone in cuts of two to serve.

When I started CrossFit, my eating habits were no better. I was a student for the first two years and ate from wherever was closest to the library, which was almost always the Chinese food truck. Or I'd take a gallon of milk to where I'd study and drink that over the course of a late-night study session. Either way, I'd feel like garbage afterward.

Even when I began to take training a little more seriously, I didn't have the organization or the cooking skills to eat consistently. Some days, it'd be two in the afternoon and I'd realize that I hadn't had a meal all day, so I'd leave the gym and binge so much food that I couldn't work out for another hour. Then I'd get home and heat up a Hungry-Man Salisbury Steak TV dinner and chase it with a pint of Ben & Jerry's. Typically, I'd still be at such a caloric deficit that I'd have to gorge again at one in the morning.

Crust

25 Oreos

4 tablespoons butter, melted

Filling

8 ounces cream cheese, softened

1 cup creamy peanut butter

$^3/_4$ cup powdered sugar

8 ounces Cool Whip

2 cups peanut butter cups, chopped

1. Preheat the oven to 350°F.
2. Make the crust. Place the cookies in the bowl of a food processor. Pulse to a fine-crumb consistency. While the processor is running, pour the melted butter into the feed chute.
3. Press the cookie crumbs into the bottom of a pie pan. Bake the crust for 5 to 7 minutes. Let the crust cool completely.
4. Make the filling. In the bowl of a stand mixer, beat the cream cheese and peanut butter until smooth. Add the powdered sugar and mix until just combined. Lastly, add the Cool Whip until just combined.
5. Pour the filling into the completely cooled crust and chill for 1 to 2 hours.
6. Top with the chopped peanut butter cups. Serve.

I wish I could say that I eventually developed the cooking skills I needed to fuel my training, but that's not what happened. I used a meal service here and there, then Sammy moved in and started taking over. Even though she can't cook for you personally, definitely check out her recipes in this book, and see what she's up to on Feeding the Frasers (FeedingTheFrasers.com), where she catalogs everything she's making for me. I know it's hard to be in charge of your own nutrition, but you can do better than eating jars of peanut butter every night.

1. STRICT PRESS

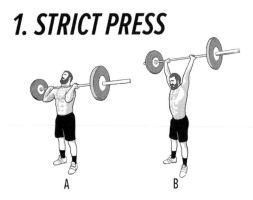

A   B

2. PUSH PRESS

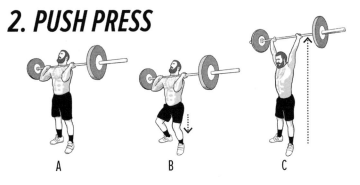

A   B   C

3. PUSH JERK

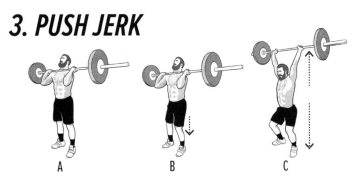

A   B   C

To Improve Your Shoulder Strength

Push Press (@ 77%)
1 × 4
4 × 5

Shoulder Press
2 sets of 10 @ 65%
2 sets of 6 @ 70%
1 set of 4 @ 75%

Shoulder Press
7 @ 68%
4 sets of 5 @ 72–75%

Push Press
4 sets of 4 reps @ 77–80%

Split Jerk
3 @ 80%
2 @ 85%
2 sets of 2 @ 80%

Seated Shoulder Press
10 mins to finish 5 reps
4 × 4 @ 85%

WORKOUT: *Deadstop Bench Presses*

5 Sets
4 Deadstop Bench Presses

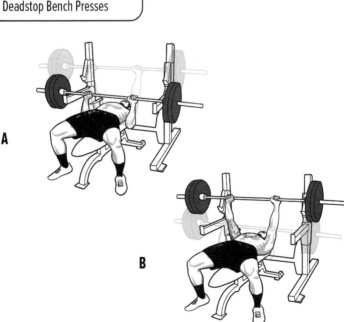

A

B

3 Sets
30 sec plank
30 sec mountain climbers
30 sec extended plank
30 sec max V-ups
Rest: 90 secs

EMOM for 10 mins
35 sec plank with dumbbell side
   pull
20 sec L-sit hold rings

To Improve Your Olympic Lifts

Hang Power Snatch
5 × 3 @ 75%

Snatch Balance
3 @ 80%
2 @ 90%
2 @ 85%
2 × 3 @ 80%

Power Snatch
3 @ 80%
2 @ 85%
1 @ 90%
2 @ 85%
3 × 2 @ 80%

Squat Snatch
1 × 3 @ 75%
2 × 3 @ 80%
2 × 1 @ 82%
1 × 3 @ 75 %

Snatch Balance
2 @ 80–85%

Clean and Jerk
7 @ 60%
Rest: 3 mins
1 @ 75%
1 @ 80%
1 @ 85
2 sets of 1 @ 75%

Clean and Jerk
1 @ 85%
2 × 2 @ 80%
1 × 2 @ 75%

EMOM for 10 mins
1 clean and jerk @ 85%

To Improve Your Deadlift

Deadlift

8 @ 45%

6 @ 55%

6 @ 65%

3 sets of 6 @ 70–72%

Deadlift

8 @ 45%

6 @ 55%

5 @ 65%

5 @ 75%

3 sets of 5 @ 80%

5 @ 75%

1 set until form breaks down
  @ 65%

Deadlift

8 @ 45%

6 @ 55%

6 @ 65%

5 @ 70%

2 sets of 5 @ 75%

Deadlift every 3 mins

1 × 7 @ 72%

1 × 6 @ 75%

3 × 5 @ 77%

Deadlift

1 × 5 @ 75%

1 × 4 @ 77%

1 × 3 @ 80%

3 × 3 @ 82–87%

Deadlift

1 × 5 @ 80%

4 × 4 @ 82–87%

**Accumulate 5 mins at top of
  Deadlift with (M 135 lbs/
  W 95 lbs)**

Hex Bar Deadlift

4 sets of 4 @ 67%

To Improve Your Squats

Back Squat
3 sets of 7 reps @ 80%

Back Squat
6 × 2 @ 85%

Overhead Squat
4 × 4 tempo @ 70%

Back Squat
6 × 6 @ 80%

Overhead Squat
1 × 4 @ 77%
1 × 4 @ 80%
1 × 3 @ 85%
1 × 1 @ 90%
1 × 1 @ 95%

Back Squat
3 × 3 @ 95%

Front Squat
1 × 1 @ 80%
3 × 8 @ 70%

Overhead Squat
4 × 3 @ 84–87%

3RM Back Squat
3 sets of 7 reps @ 80%

Overhead Squat
Every 90 secs for 6 sets
Sets 1–2: 3 @ 80%
Sets 3–4: 3 @ 85%
Sets 5–6: 4 @ 75%

2

Endurance

It wasn't like I didn't know I had no engine in the run-up to the 2013 Regionals. I just didn't have the motivation to fix it. So instead of doing all the workouts Jade would program for me, I'd cherry-pick whatever I was already good at or go deadlift with the cute girl who asked me to train with her. My strength alone got me to Regionals, and I had no expectation of making it to the Games anyway. So why not work out how I wanted to?

I was feeling especially confident after "Jackie," the first workout of Regionals and the one where I'd lagged on the rower and then screamed through the 45-pound thrusters. I expected to follow that pattern for the rest of the competition—fall behind on the cardio parts and then use my strength to overcome the deficit. That'd be no problem, right?

Obviously not. I had no aerobic capacity, so I'd get into trouble no matter how "light" the weight was. *Okay,* I'd tell myself. *It's okay. Just sit here for a minute until your lungs don't hurt anymore and then get going.* Using that strategy on one event, I got 18th place and practically crawled off the floor.

Nothing makes you aware of the corners you're cutting more than being the last guy at the end of a workout, especially doing movements that are normally light enough to be a warm-up for you. And that wasn't the last time I would be humbled that weekend. Even though I had some standout performances at Regionals—including a three-rep overhead squat at 315 pounds—I fell apart whenever the breathing got heavy.

On the drive back to Vermont, the lesson was clear: If I wanted to even think about using my strength, I had to build a foundation of endurance. I did that by mastering three movements—rowing, running, and swimming—and that's when I started to fall in love with CrossFit, when I realized that I had the power to identify a weakness, modify my training, and improve it. It fundamentally changed how I competed, and I'll show you how to do the same.

Endurance 101

Before Regionals in 2013, I'd started lifting at Champlain Valley but refused to try a "real" CrossFit workout. I'd mess around with the weightlifting workouts, like Heavy Grace, but never anything with even a hint of cardio. I'd done a sport where you rest for minutes in between sets, so why would I want to run or row or get on a bike at all, let alone between the other movements?

It sounded miserable, and when I finally got talked into doing a METCON (metabolic conditioning) of kettlebell swings and running, it was just as bad as I'd expected.

I could do the swings as quickly as humanly possible. I knew

KETTLEBELL SWING TECHNIQUE

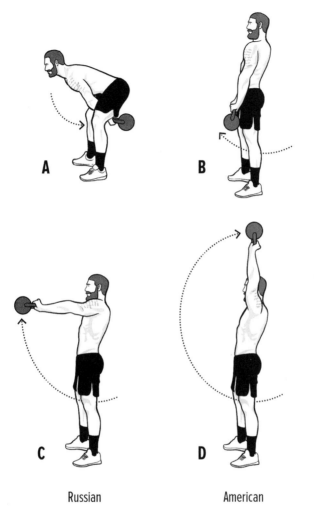

Russian   American

from Olympic lifting how to hinge forward and hike the bell behind me, then how to stand up and thrust my hips forward to
get it above my head. I finished those sets well before everyone

else—but they all caught me on the run. In fact, it looked like some of them even recovered a bit as they jogged past me. How was that possible?

It was hard to understand at first. Time had just never been crucial to my success before. Yeah, you had to finish your Olympic lift within the 60 seconds, but I could pump my hips 20 times and still make that cutoff. So having to complete a workout as quickly as possible was similar to adding an entirely new field to the scorecard, like a dance contest after the snatch and clean and jerk at an Olympic weightlifting meet. I could learn to do it eventually, but it would take a long time.

EXERCISE: *Rowing Drills*

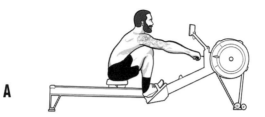

A

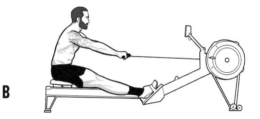

B

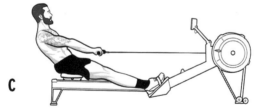

C

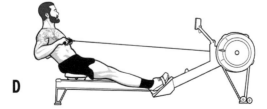

D

It all started with rowing, probably the most common cardio movement in our sport. Not every box has a fleet of Assault Bikes or SkiErgs, but they'll usually have a wall of Concept2s, which is how I began my endurance journey. After the 2013 Regionals, I committed to rowing 5,000 meters every day for a year to build my engine and learn the proper technique, which actually has a lot in common with snatching.

You start by pushing with the legs, and when they're straight and tapped out, you open your hips. Once your hips are opened up, that's when you follow through and pull with your arms. Just like with Olympic lifting, you have to finish one stage of the movement before you can go on to the next. But even though I was familiar with that concept, I still had to break down the movement into its parts and practice.

ARMS ONLY

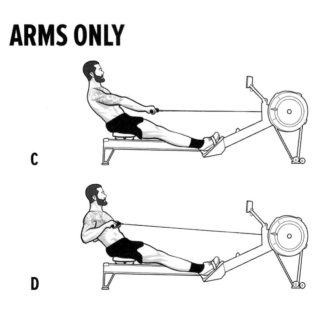

C

D

Let's start with the end of the stroke: the arm pull. In this first drill, have your knees slightly bent and use your back muscles to pull the handle into your body. Your arms should be straight to start, and at the end your shoulder blades should be pinched together.

In the next drill, keep your arms straight and lean your torso forward and then pull it backward. Once you're leaning back (you should feel your abs engaged), begin the arm pull you practiced in the last drill.

ARMS AND BODY

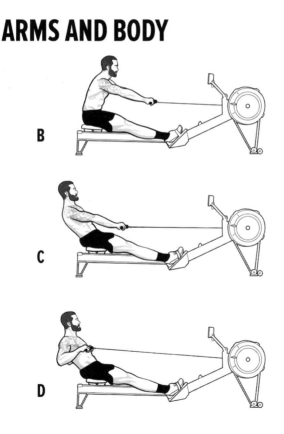

Then you're ready for the most important step: the leg drive. For this last drill, keep your torso still and your arms relaxed, and use the heels of your feet to push away from the rower. This is how you generate the majority of your power, and you want to use every last bit of energy in your legs before leaning back and initiating the arm pull. It seems simple, but it took me hundreds of hours to master.

LEGS ONLY

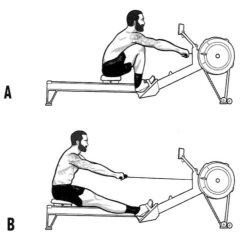

A

B

WORKOUT: *The Fraser Row Camp (Lite)*

Row 2,000 meters daily for 2 weeks

During the year I was rowing every day, I lived in the basement of my parents' house, which was a tiny one-bedroom and had low ceilings and no windows. I loved it down there. Especially after I qualified for the Games and had to ramp up my training, I never had to worry about paying rent, collecting my mail, or fighting with the landlords about the sound of barbells crashing in the tiny 175-square-foot gym I'd created.

At first it was hard to do rowing intervals in what was basically my living room. But gradually I learned how to flip the switch from hanging out to training time, and that small, dark space became the place where I looked forward to suffering, even in June, when it was easily 100 degrees and all I had was a box fan that barely moved the air.

Lucky for you, I'm suggesting that you row 2,000 meters every day for only two weeks, and I encourage you to do what I did and break it up differently each day: 4 sets of 500 one day, sprint intervals of 100 meters the next. Also, experiment with the settings on the damper (the lever on the side of the circular flywheel at the front of the rower). The higher the damper number, the more difficult each stroke is, and the farther you go with each pull.

Because every person (and every workout) is different, there's no right answer as to where you should set yours, but I've practiced at the highest and lowest and everything in between to know how they all feel.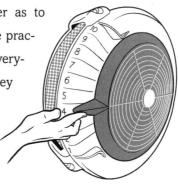

Once you've mastered the damper, you can move on to more advanced techniques.

WORKOUT: *TABATA Rowing*

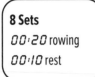

8 Sets

00:20 rowing

00:10 rest

Now it's time to play around with other variables, like the foot stretcher. Generally, the foot strap should go around the widest part of your foot.

If you're constantly getting on and off the rower, you may want to leave the straps loose to cut down on the time spent transitioning (which is something I recommend you practice).

There's also a hack to get an extra calorie off your first pull if you're using a Concept2 rower. It's probably not the one you've heard of, 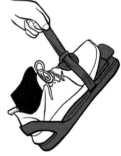 where you start with a quarter-pull, half-pull, and three-quarter pull as quickly as possible. The more effective way is to take the handle out of the cradle and get all the way to the very front of the rower. Then explode backward with the biggest, longest pull you can, to your chin if it's possible. After that, straighten your arms without moving your torso and do another quick, tiny pull. To recap: the most powerful, overexaggerated stroke you've got and then another one that's around a foot long.

Knowing the equipment you use is essential to success, and those two strokes should get you around two calories. That's a huge advantage if you're doing something short, like a rowing Tabata. But it's probably not worth the effort if you're doing, say, a marathon row.

A quick explanation about the CrossFit Games, which are unlike any other major sporting event in the world. For starters, you have no idea what, exactly, is going to be programmed, so you have to make educated guesses based off the venue, terrain, and past workouts.

There's always a decent number of "pure" CrossFit workouts—a few rounds of two or three movements that should last between 7 and 20 minutes total. There's also always a run, a swim, and a strength event, like a one-rep max or a lift "ladder," where you have to hit progressively heavier weights. And there's always at least one "named" workout, classic benchmarks that are well-known in the community, and which most of the spectators have also done. And then there are years when totally new equipment is introduced, like the Pig and the pegboard in 2015.

Other than knowing those general guidelines, you're more or less shooting blind for the majority of the 15 or so workouts that come up. Sometimes we find out the details of an event the night before. Other times, we get only a few minutes. In 2018, we had to do a workout called "Chaos," where we didn't know anything, not even the rep scheme or what the next movement in the workout would be. You just had to watch the competitors ahead of you or wait for your judge to raise her hand, which meant that you were five reps away from finishing that exercise and moving on. I didn't love that event. I thought it was less about testing fitness and more about rewarding the person who guessed the time domain correctly, but that's part of competition. You accept it and move on.

Regardless of the events that are programmed each year, they're all tested ahead of time by athletes who were on the cusp of qualifying but didn't make it. Many are designed so that barely anyone finishes—or maybe even no one at all. That can make it very difficult to pace yourself, especially when you're doing a workout you've never done before, you're jacked up on adrenaline, and you're right next to nine of your biggest competitors. So even though every professional athlete says that their sport is just as mental as it is physical, that's doubly true in CrossFit.

However, another big difference between us and other sports is the scoring system. You don't have to win every event. In fact, in 2016, the first year that I became a CrossFit champion, I won only one of the 15 events. Consistency beats specialization every time, which is why I'm always saying that I train my weaknesses. Those are what determine your placement at the Games, not your strengths.

WORKOUT: *Half-Marathon Row*

Row 21,097 meters

Looking back, I'm so grateful I didn't qualify for the Games in 2013. If I'd gotten out to California and been told that I had to row a half marathon on the very first day, I would've walked right out. I knew there was no way I was going to win, and you want me to sit on a rower for 90 minutes?

I was more psychologically and physically prepared when a marathon row came up again in 2018, but I wildly underestimated how much I'd have to hydrate during the 42,195 meters. I brought eight liters of water with me but figured I'd only drink two, and I finished it all with 17,000 meters left. And then I really started to sweat.

They'd told us during the athlete briefing that we couldn't piss on the rower, and the HQ team was convinced that I'd broken that rule. Most of the athletes had two puddles on either side of the rower from where sweat would drip off their elbows, but I had a pool that covered two and a half feet in every direction. Coincidentally, I was also next to where a set of rowers' cables was plugged in, and I found out later that they had an emergency meeting to discuss what they'd do if my sweat puddle short-circuited the machines.

While I was rowing, though, I wasn't concerned about the electricity. I was worried that I'd overheat, cramp up, and have to withdraw, especially after I misjudged just how long a marathon would take. With 17,000 meters left, I thought I was in the home stretch, only to realize that meant I had 34 500s left to row. To try to limit my sweating, I dropped the pace from 1:50 to 2:00, which meant I still had another hour of rowing left. My throat was dry. My ass was sore. My puddle kept growing.

The Mat from 2013 would've quit a half hour in, but I pushed through and took 11th with a time of two hours and 48 minutes. It was my worst performance at that year's Games, but the one I had worked the hardest to achieve, and afterward I took rowing off my mental list of weaknesses. It was by no means a strength, but I had other endurance skills I needed to work on.

CrossFit Endurance

WORKOUT: *The Zone Two Test*

> 90-minute bike ride in Zone Two (85–89% of your lactate threshold)

Building your aerobic foundation might not feel like work at all. In 2017, I went to the Sports Medicine and Performance Center at the University of Colorado to learn more about the physiology behind my workouts. As part of the evaluation, they tested my lactic threshold by having me run on a treadmill that got half a mile faster every three minutes. All the way through minute 39, I felt great, good enough to go for hours—but as soon as they turned it up one more notch, I knew almost immediately that I wouldn't make it to the next interval, and I didn't.

To explain why I fell off the cliff so hard, they showed me a graph of the lactic acid in my body, and the line spiked right at minute 39, when lactic acid was being produced at a faster rate than it could be cleared out. At that point, my body did everything it could to shut me down, and the takeaway was obvious: Do everything you can to raise the lactic threshold by spending more time at moderate intensity, also called "Zone Two."

How I trained changed completely. Up until that point, I would sit on a bike for 90 minutes maybe once a season, and more to say that I'd done it than anything else. After that test, I'd train at Zone Two about three times a week.

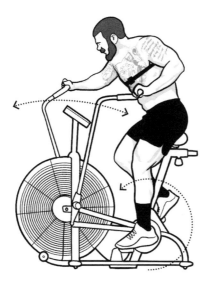

Your heart rate for Zone Two training will be different from mine. To find yours, you first need to know your functional threshold power (FTP), the highest effort you can sustain for one hour, as measured in watts on a stationary bike. However, according to my endurance coach, Chris Hinshaw, you don't have to ride for a full hour. Instead, pedal for just 20 minutes at the greatest intensity you can maintain the entire time. At the end, you'll have two numbers: a wattage and a heart rate. Take 95 percent of that and it's your FTP. The optimal Zone Two is 55 to 75 percent of that wattage and 70 to 83 percent of that heart rate.

For example, let's say you averaged 284 watts and a heart rate of 166 in your 20-minute ride. If you take 95 percent of that, the estimate for your FTP is 270 watts and a threshold heart rate of 158. Therefore, your optimal Zone Two training range is 149 to 203 watts (55 percent to 75 percent) and a heart rate of 111 to 131 beats per minute (70 percent to 83 percent). That's probably more math than you were expecting, but optimizing your fitness isn't as straightforward as it may seem.

Just because a workout is really, really hard doesn't necessarily mean that you're getting better. But if you devote the time to improving your endurance, eventually it will become something that you can fall back on no matter what the workout is.

WORKOUT: *Run, Swim, Run*

Run 1.5 miles
Swim 500 meters
Run 1.5 miles

Before we cover proper running technique, I want to emphasize again the importance of having confidence in your cardio.

At the 2017 Games, Ricky Garard was leading the first leg of the run-swim-run. I didn't know then that he was taking performance-enhancing drugs, which he'd be caught and suspended for afterward, but I did know that he was a phenomenal runner and a terrible swimmer. If he hit the water after a 5:30 mile pace, he'd be completely recovered, and the swim wouldn't be long enough for me to catch up before he'd lose me on the second run. But if I pushed him closer to a 5:20 pace on that first run, he might panic when he hit the water. We'd both be hurting, but I trusted my recovery more than his.

While we were on the first run, I worked my way to the front of the pack and started egging on Garard. *Come on, man,* I said. *Let's go faster. There we go. We can pull away from the entire group.* I'd draft off him for a bit and then pass him if I felt like he was slowing down. Every time, he'd speed up to catch me.

It was a risky strategy but paid off. He burned too bright, couldn't recover, and finished that event in 12th.

I didn't break any records—I got 7th—but here I was, someone who could barely do five burpees in a row a few years earlier, literally running toward the water knowing that I'd hit it gasping for air. And I did it with no hesitation. I slipped my shoes off and my goggles on, and dove into the lake without breaking my stride. This is why endurance is so important. It allows you to control the flow of the workout and stay cool if something unexpected happens.

So if all you want to do is build your cardio foundation, running and rowing are great ways to do it, and you can stop here. But if you're looking to become the best athlete you can, you're going to have to train how others won't.

Endurance for Competitive Athletes

WORKOUT: *The Beach*

> Swim 250 yards

You may be wondering why I'm including swimming here. After all, there's never more than one swimming event at the Games, so why focus on something that's so rare? Careful. There's a big difference between something that's low-probability and something that's low-frequency. Yes, there's *only* one swim event, but there's *always* one swim event. We know it's going to show up, and if you want to have any future as a competitive CrossFit athlete, there's no excuse for coming unprepared. That's the mistake I made three years in a row.

A lake is not an ocean. I hope that's obvious to you, but it took me a long time to fully understand, so I'll say it again. Just because you aren't afraid of drowning in the lake where you grew up doesn't mean you aren't going to panic when you dive into the surf of a 500-yard open water swim off the coast of California. And on a July day in 2014, during the first event of the first day of my first CrossFit Games, I panicked almost immediately.

Up until that point, I thought I'd cracked the code on how to be a competitive CrossFit athlete. A few months earlier, I'd won Regionals, with an average event placement of 2.5 out of 45 men, and I thought I'd prepared enough to do well at the Games, if not win it all. Now I can see that there were gaps in my training that year that were as big as Lake Champlain, and on my short list of priorities, swimming wasn't even an afterthought.

I'd never tried to swim as part of a longer workout, and after I sprinted along the beach and crashed into the ocean, I couldn't breathe. No, it was more than that. I couldn't even convince myself to put my face in the water and start to freestyle. Instead, I sidestroked the entire time and came in 17th place with a time of 36:31, about seven minutes slower than the guy who won.

I wish I could tell you that I committed myself to training that weakness during the following season, but you already know that's not true.

WORKOUT: *Pier Paddle*

> Swim 500 yards
> (in open water if possible)

I was able to take second place overall at the Games in 2014 by putting not that much effort into my training (and working a full-time summer internship in the months leading up to the competition). That level of success was exciting. I still planned on graduating from UVM and getting a job in engineering, and here was this crazy thing I could tell my co-workers that I'd done. After the 2014 champion retired, I was even more stoked. If he wasn't around the following year, who was next in line? It had to be me.

On that first day of competition in 2015, at least I could say that I'd practiced swimming, but not in open water, and definitely not with any kind of coherent plan. Instead, I'd swim 50 meters in the pool, rest until my heart rate was almost back to resting, and swim another 50 meters. I thought I was practicing correctly, but yet again I ended up sidestroking the entire race and finished in 12th.

It was the same story in 2016—but worse. My aerobic foundation was better, and I was finally comfortable enough to sink my face in the water and take proper strokes, so I placed higher. But that was more due to luck than my own preparation.

Up until a few weeks before the Games, I didn't even get into the pool, and even then the longest I ever swam was 200 meters. Plus I wouldn't flip turn, so I was basically cheating by catching the wall and getting in two breaths every time I switched directions. Yet somehow I was still surprised when I got into the ocean that year and it felt totally different from the pool. I'd take a few halfhearted strokes, but whenever I lost sight of the course buoys, I'd take it as an excuse to pop my head out, get in a couple big breaths, then keep going.

But that was it. After years of phoning it in, I finally decided to train swimming as seriously as I trained everything else, and it started off with yet another lesson in humility.

WORKOUT: *Kick Work*

Kick only
300 kick, long fins, 1 min rest
2 × 100 kick, no fins, 1 min rest
300 kick, long fins, 1 min rest
4 × 50 kick, no fins, 45 sec rest
300 kick, long fins, 1 min rest
8 × 25 kick, no fins, 30 sec rest
300 kick, long fins, 30 sec rest

At the Sports Medicine and Performance Center, the same place where I got my lactic threshold tested, they put me in a tank with cameras mounted at the front, sides, and bottom of the pool. Before I swam, they showed me a video of what your stroke should

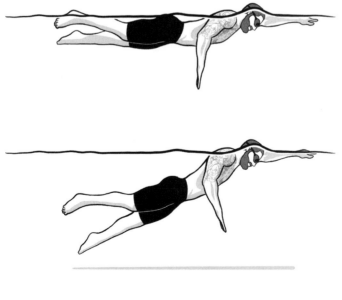

WORKOUT: *Learn to Kick*

> **10 Sets**
> 25-meter Freestyle Kicking with one leg
> Stationary Kicking with your body vertical

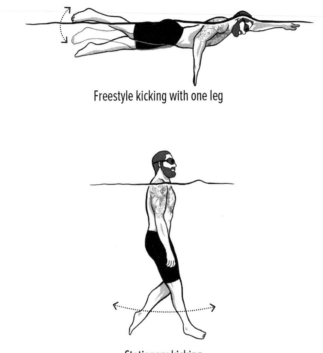

Freestyle kicking with one leg

Stationary kicking

look like: your hips on the surface of the water and your body in one vertical line. After I swam for a minute, they showed me a video of what it shouldn't look like: your hips dragging in the water so low that your toes scrape the bottom of the tank three feet below you.

I watched that second video for a dozen seconds and then had a realization—this wasn't an instructional video. It was me on a 30-second delay. I truly felt like my entire body was floating on the surface, and I was shocked that my body awareness could be so off.

Learning how to stay on top of the water required me to fix everything else that was wrong with my stroke. And there was a lot wrong.

The first area to improve? My kick. I'd been bending my knees, not moving my legs from the hips, which created drag on the water, slowed me down, and caused me to sink. I also wasn't exhaling when my face was in the pool—I'd try to both exhale

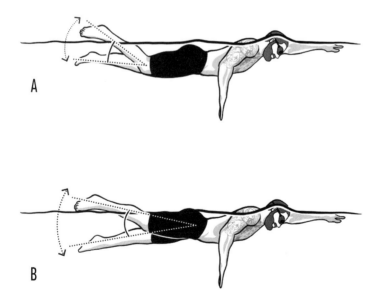

and inhale every time I came up for a breath—which made my torso even more buoyant than my lower body. Like a metal plow, I dragged through the water.

Eventually, I addressed those problems and moved on to the next weakness: my stroke. Up to that point, my thinking was that you want to be as streamlined as possible when you swim, right? So I'd reach right above my head and then pull my arms underneath my body so that I was even narrower than my shoulders. Needless to say, that's not at all what you want.

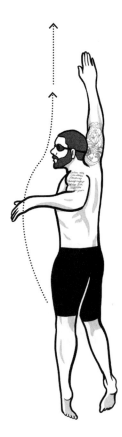

You want your arms to be a bit wider than your hips, but it took me months to make the correction. Back when I was lifting with Coach Polakowski, if he pointed out some flaw in my lifting technique, I could almost always feel it and fix it. But something about being in the water totally messed me up.

Like I did with the row, I broke down the movement and focused on each tiny component. I used paddles on my hands so I could better feel the sensation of grabbing the water. I put buoys between my feet so I didn't have to worry about my kick. And I did something I hadn't even known was possible: train my breathing muscles.

CrossFit Games Endurance

WORKOUT: *POWERbreathe Protocool*

> 30 inhalations daily
> for 5 weeks

I knew of Chris Hinshaw long before I met him in person. After I got thrashed in the sprinting events at the 2015 Games, I was trying to cobble together running workouts, and a friend passed along what he was doing for speed and endurance. It all came from Hinshaw, who's done 10 Ironman triathlons and coached 40 podium Games athletes.

His programming was brilliant, and I knew I wanted to meet him face-to-face, so I signed up for one of his Aerobic Capacity seminars. Afterward, I approached him and pulled out a wad of his workouts, which I'd folded and stuffed in my back pocket. I didn't know how he'd react, but in typical Hinshaw fashion, he had a million thoughts on how I could improve, and we've worked together ever since.

It's indisputable that Hinshaw knows his stuff, but I still didn't believe him when he said I wasn't breathing right. I had a pretty good engine by this point, so my lungs had to be decent, you know? Wrong again. I made that realization one day when we were doing a workout in the pool, and it felt like the pressure of the water on my chest was suffocating me. The only way I could breathe was if I got my torso out of the pool completely.

It turns out that my diaphragm and intercostal muscles, which run between the ribs and help you contract your lungs, weren't strong enough to allow me to breathe at high intensities, hence the drowning feeling. To compensate, they'd recruit blood from my arms and legs, making it even harder to finish the swim sets. Hinshaw would never say "I told you so," but he'd told me so.

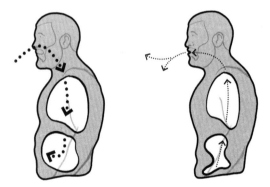

Hard Work Pays Off

Based on his advice, I started doing the POWERbreathe protocol. I'd breathe in quickly, deeply, and forcefully, then breathe out slowly and gently. I did this for 30 breaths every night and saw that my engine was better after about five weeks. At the same time, we also worked on maintaining the same breathing rhythm even when I was tired. If your brain can predict when it'll get its next hit of oxygen, the whole body relaxes and you end up using less energy.

WORKOUT: *Stroke, Buoy, Stroke*

Swim 1 mile

After I had fixed my swimming technique and my breathing pattern, all that was left was practicing, and I swam more during the 2020 season than in the rest of my CrossFit career combined. We'd be in the water twice, sometimes three times, a week year-round.

I was especially lucky to train alongside Tia-Clair Toomey-Orr, the five-time women's CrossFit champion and one of the best swimmers in the sport, but I'd have trouble sleeping the night before our sessions. I was nervous, and driving over to the lake in the morning, I'd have a pit in my stomach as we crossed the bridge and I saw the buoys that Shane, her husband and the coach for both of us, had set up for the day. When we got into the water, it always felt twice as long as it'd looked from the car, and it looked pretty long.

We didn't add any other movements to the swim workouts for the first few months of the 2020 season, and those days were almost unbearably boring. Because we were in a lake, you didn't even have lines to look at like you do at the bottom of a pool, so the view never changed, especially not for the half hour it'd take us to swim the mile. You'd stare at the brown water, stroke, stroke, pop your head up, and see the buoy. Then it'd be more brown water, stroke, stroke.

But all that hard work paid off. Swimming is one of the events that Noah Ohlsen beat me in during the 2019 Games, and it could've been the reason I lost the entire competition if there had been a different top-ten configuration that year. But in 2020, I beat him and took second in the pool event, which is a good lesson if you hope to become an elite competitor: train for everything. And once you're physically prepared, you can focus on the mental side of endurance.

The Endurance Mentality

JOURNAL ENTRY—What's the discomfort that you fear most? Is it the long, slow grind of a 35-minute chipper? Is it the fire breathing of an all-out sprint? Is it during barbell cycling? Sprint intervals? Bodyweight squats that you know could be faster but burn like hell? Identify the type of workout or movement that you most dread and explain why.

It's easy to think of endurance as a marathon row or an ocean swim, but to endure really means one thing to me—sacrificing a moment of pain for a lifetime of freedom. That's what I've been able to achieve with my CrossFit career, but that wasn't my mindset during the 2014 and 2015 seasons. Even though I thought I might have the potential to be the best, I was scared.

During those two years, I made it well known that I finished a pint of Ben & Jerry's ice cream every night. At the time, I told myself that was the reward for a day of hard training, but looking back now, I see that I was just making excuses. If I didn't end up winning the Games, I could say it was because of my eating. Or because the events were unfair. Or because I didn't really care about CrossFit in the first place. None of those was true, but like I said, I was scared to fully invest myself.

So after I lost in 2015, did I want to cut my losses and move on from CrossFit, like I'd done with Olympic lifting, or commit myself without these safety nets? I opted for the latter—but that's not what I'm going to recommend for you, at least not now.

Before we move on to the larger questions about whether you want to be the CrossFit Games champion, I want you to start simple and think about physical pain. Where does it get spiciest in a workout for you? When do you want to quit most? Once you can identify the sticking points in your training, you can work to address them.

WORKOUT: *Seven Minutes in Heaven*

> **As many as possible**
> *7:00* Burpees

It sounds corny to say, but there's also a difference between pain and discomfort, and I've felt plenty of both to know. Pain is when you've snapped one of the wings off a vertebra in your spine, and you're one bad lift away from a slipped disc and a life of limited mobility. Pain is your body telling you that something is seriously wrong. There have been times I've had to push through pain, like when I tore my LCL at the Games, but more often than not, what you're experiencing is discomfort. That doesn't mean it hurts any less, but at least you know it's going to end after the workout (or maybe five or ten minutes after that).

Pain is dangerous. Discomfort is where you get better. That's not all it takes, but you can't keep improving in this sport without it. So, sorry, CrossFit never becomes easy. You just learn to handle the discomfort better, which is why I like this workout of seven minutes of burpees. Because burpees are a low-impact body-weight exercise, you're probably going to experience discomfort, not pain. Still, your whole body will be lit up, which makes this a good place to start if you want to be able to endure a moment of pain for a lifetime of freedom.

WORKOUT: *A Lactic Acid Machine*

8 Rounds
Assault Bike Tabata
00:20 on
00:10 off

Another way to lean deep into the discomfort is on the Assault Bike, which Hinshaw explained to me like this: It's a machine specifically designed to create fatigue. Your legs generate lactic acid, and your arms generate lactic acid, and the lactic acid overloads those muscles and eventually hits the bloodstream and circulates through your entire body. Especially if you're doing a Tabata, there's no way you'll be able to clear the lactic out during the ten seconds of rest, so it'll build and build.

If you do this workout right, be careful getting off because you might collapse directly onto the ground. As much as you won't want to, also try to walk around to get the circulation going.

More likely than not, you'll never want to get on the Assault Bike again, but you've got to fight that urge for two reasons. First, you can use the bike to build your capacity in your legs by training just your legs, without the additional lactic from your arms. And vice versa. Second, it can improve your running. I run between 175 and 180 steps per minute, which equates to 90 revolutions per minute on the bike. Once I started training at 90 rpm, my work on the bike translated to my work on the track—though I still had to bury myself on the track.

WORKOUT: *The Mile Finisher*

1 × 600-meter sprint
2 × 400-meter sprints
2 × 200-meter sprints
2 × 100-meter sprints
Mile time trial

This was one of the most brutal and surprising workouts I ever did with Hinshaw.

It started with 2,000 meters broken down into sprint intervals. Hinshaw is never overgenerous with his rests, so I was huffing and puffing by the end. Then he told me that I had to run three kilometers, but with a catch: The final mile of the 3K had to be 5:20 or under.

That's impossible, I told him. He didn't say a word. *Can I rest before we do the 3K?* No. *Can I rest before I do that final mile?* Also no. If I were deep into an endurance event, he told me, I had to know that I could do the thing that we'd talked about but never put into practice: breaking the rubber band between me and my competitor.

It would go something like this (at least in theory): Another guy and I are out at the front of the pack, and we're each gunning for that 100-point event win. So how do I shake him? Well, if I put enough distance between us, even for just a few seconds, the gap would seem insurmountable to him. He'd decide

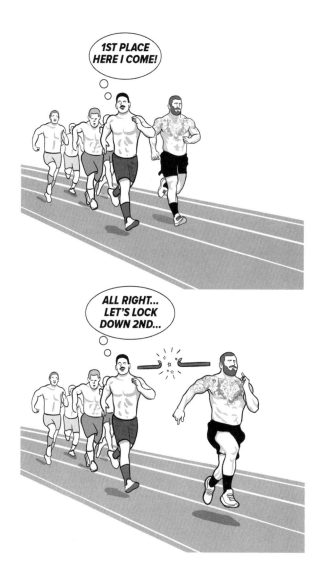

that, instead of trying to catch up to me, it would be better to stay ahead of the pack and protect his second-place finish. Once that psychological shift happened, from chasing me to avoiding getting caught by the rest of the field, the mental rubber band between us would be broken and the race would be mine, as I'd soon find out.

Against truly every one of my expectations, I hit that 5:20 mile. It wasn't pretty, but it gave me confidence a few months later at the 2016 Games. The first event was a 7-kilometer trail run, and Josh Bridges and I were out in front. Naturally, we throttled back a bit because we were far enough ahead that no one was likely to catch us. In 2014 or 2015, I would've grunted it out with him until the end and tried to outsprint him at the finish. But this time was different.

I was a little ahead of Bridges, and when I saw a corner at the top of the hill we were running up, I knew what to do. As soon as I turned it, I sprinted as hard as I could. When Bridges next saw me, I was gone, too far gone for him to catch me. Or at least that's what he thought. I was actually so winded from the sprint that I could barely keep jogging, but breaking the rubber band worked. I won the race by almost 90 seconds.

Winning the trail run would've seemed impossible three years earlier, as I was doing my first Open workout and Jade was screaming at me to get up off the floor and finish the three burpees I had left in the workout, or when I was so winded at Regionals that I could barely breathe. But now, while everyone else had been caught in bottlenecks and dust clouds in the backwoods, I had taken the lead, dropped the hammer, and never looked back on the trail run.

Hard Work Pays Off

Eating for Endurance

I have to eat constantly throughout the day. I know that sounds like a lot of people's fantasy, but trust me, when it's 6 p.m. and you just finished your third workout of the day and still have two hours of mobility to do, another meal feels like a chore. Sammy knows this, so she's constantly feeding me, whether it's having my second breakfast ready when I walk in the door or putting a cut apple in front of me while I scroll through Instagram. If you want to train at a high intensity, you have to stay fueled constantly, so here are a few recipes that are quick to eat in between sessions.

Granola

$^1/_4$ cup pistachios

$^1/_4$ cup pepitas

$^1/_4$ cup hazelnuts

2 cups gluten-free rolled oats

2 teaspoons flaky salt

2 teaspoons cinnamon

$^1/_2$ cup almond butter

$^1/_4$ cup maple syrup

$^1/_4$ cup coconut oil

$^1/_4$ cup golden raisins (or dried fruit of choice!)

1. Preheat the oven to 300°F.
2. Rough chop the pistachios, pepitas, and hazelnuts. In a large bowl, mix the nuts with the oats, salt, and cinnamon.
3. In a separate small bowl, combine the almond butter, maple syrup, and coconut oil. Microwave in 15-second intervals until the oil is melted and mix the ingredients together until smooth.
4. Pour the wet ingredients into the large bowl containing the nuts and oats. Mix well to fully incorporate.
5. Lay out the granola on a large baking sheet and shake gently to evenly distribute. Gently pat down with the back side of a spatula.
6. Bake for 15 minutes. Remove from the oven, toss the granola, and gently pat down into a smooth single layer (this will help it clump together!).

7. Bake for an additional 15 minutes. Remove from the oven, add the dried fruit on top, and cool completely (roughly 40 to 60 minutes) to allow the granola to clump together. Enjoy.

I'm not a morning person. Especially during the pandemic, when Tia and I were more or less inseparable from sunup to sundown, she had to give me an hour or so to wake up in the morning before we could start joking around, let alone training. If you're a serious CrossFit athlete, you probably have to wake up early, whether it's to coach the 5 a.m. class or to get that day's first session under your belt before work. However, that's no excuse to skip a meal. Even though you may be half asleep when you walk out the door, you at least need something in your bag for immediately after you finish.

Sourdough Sprout Sandwich

$^1/_2$ avocado, sliced

2 slices sourdough bread, toasted

2 tablespoons chive cream cheese

$^1/_4$ cup alfalfa sprouts

4 ounces deli chicken breast

1. Lay the slices of avocado on one slice of toasted sourdough.
2. Spread the chive cream cheese on the other slice of toasted sourdough.
3. Top the avocado with sprouts and then the chicken slices. Close the sandwich with the slice of sourdough spread with cream cheese.
4. Cut and enjoy.

It's also crucial that you get outside the gym occasionally. During the 2020 season, I was able to do a few workouts with Sammy, which are some of my fondest memories from that year—in retrospect. At the time, they were barbaric. We had to sprint up a hill that was a half-mile long and at a 40-degree angle. One of us was wearing a vest (it wasn't Sammy), and there was no shade anywhere around. I'd do one more ascent than Sammy, so we'd usually end at around the same time, and I've never been more ready for a thousand gallons of water and some light sandwiches.

Huli Huli Hot Party Wings

3 pounds chicken wings

1 teaspoon salt

1 teaspoon smoked paprika

1 teaspoon ground cumin

2 teaspoons garlic powder

Pinch of cayenne

1 cup pineapple juice

$^{1}/_{3}$ cup ketchup

$^{1}/_{4}$ cup tamari (or soy sauce)

3 tablespoons Mike's Hot Honey, divided

1 tablespoon ginger juice

2 teaspoons garlic, grated

1 teaspoon red wine vinegar

Pinch of red pepper flakes

$^{1}/_{2}$ cup plain Greek yogurt

$^{1}/_{2}$ teaspoon lemon juice

2 tablespoons cilantro, chopped, plus more for garnish

Fresno chile, sliced

1. Lay the wings on a wire rack above a baking sheet.
   Pat dry with a paper towel.
2. In a small bowl, mix the salt, smoked paprika, cumin,
   garlic powder, and cayenne. Sprinkle the wings with
   the spice mix.
3. Working in two batches, set the air fryer to 400°F.
   Cook for 20 minutes. Remove the first batch, place on
   a baking sheet, and set in the oven to keep warm while
   the second batch cooks.

4. While the wings are cooking, prepare the sauce. In a medium saucepan over medium heat, whisk the pineapple juice, ketchup, tamari, 2 tablespoons of the honey, the ginger juice, garlic, red wine vinegar, and red pepper flakes. Bring the sauce to a boil, reduce the heat to medium, and simmer for 10 to 12 minutes until the sauce thickens and has reduced by half.
5. When the second batch of wings has finished cooking, toss all the wings with the sauce and return all to the air fryer basket. Cook the sauced wings for an additional 5 minutes to caramelize.
6. Make the dipping sauce: In a small bowl, whisk the yogurt, remaining 1 tablespoon hot honey, the lemon juice, and cilantro.
7. Top the wings with additional cilantro and chilies, chilies, and serve with the zesty citrus yogurt dipping sauce.

During marathon days of training, I didn't have a lot of time at home, so it was really nice when Sammy made food I could grab and take with me to eat in the car. Other times, what I wanted was to slowly pick at a meal throughout the night. You may not always have the energy or the opportunity for a civilized sit-down with plates and napkins, so don't be afraid to eat on the go. You can ingest a lot of calories during the fifteen-minute drive from your house to the gym.

French Dip

2 teaspoons garlic powder

2 teaspoons black pepper

2 teaspoons salt, plus more for seasoning

$1^1/_2$ pounds sirloin cap

4 cups beef stock

1 sprig thyme

1 sprig rosemary

$^1/_4$ teaspoon ground pepper

2 cloves garlic

4 hoagie rolls, cut in half

8 slices provolone cheese

1. Preheat the Traeger Grill (or conventional grill/oven) to 450–500°F/230–260°C.
2. In a small bowl, mix the garlic powder, black pepper, and salt. Season the sirloin cap liberally with the rub. Place the sirloin cap on the grill and roast for 45 minutes. Reduce the grill temperature to 325°F/160°C and cook for an additional 30 minutes or until the internal temperature reaches 125°F/50°C. Remove the sirloin cap from the grill. Wrap it in foil and let it rest for 15 minutes before slicing.
3. While the sirloin cap is on the grill, prepare the au jus. Place the beef stock, thyme, rosemary, pepper, and garlic in a saucepot. Bring to a simmer for 30 to 45 minutes. Season with salt to taste and strain before serving.

4. To assemble the sandwich, place the hoagie rolls on a baking sheet, cut-side up, top each with a slice of the cheese, and warm in the oven or on the hot grill until the cheese is melted. Remove the sirloin cap from the foil and slice thinly. Add the steak slices to the sandwich and serve with a small bowl of au jus for dipping.

I haven't eaten a French dip sandwich on the C2 bike, but there are some days I've certainly thought about it, mostly during those long Zone Two sessions when I'm already watching *The Office* and zoning out. That's another good way to know if you're training at the right intensity: moving, but not too quickly.

Taquitos: Fiesta and Bacon Ranch

2 rotisserie chickens, shredded

8 ounces cream cheese

$^1/_4$ cup sour cream

8 ounces pepper jack cheese, cubed

$^1/_4$ cup green onions, chopped

2 tablespoons fajita seasoning

$^1/_4$ cup corn (canned and drained or roasted)

$^1/_4$ cup black beans, drained

2 slices bacon, chopped

2 tablespoons ranch seasoning

20 flour (or corn—CAUTION: They break as they bake) tortillas

Sour cream, salsa, guacamole, etc., for serving (optional)

1. Preheat the oven to 425°F.
2. In a large bowl, mix the shredded chicken, cream cheese, sour cream, cubed cheese, and green onions. Divide the mixture into two separate bowls.
3. For the fiesta taquito, add the fajita seasoning, corn, and beans to one bowl; for the bacon ranch taquito, add the bacon and ranch seasoning to the other bowl.
4. Spoon 2 tablespoons of the fiesta mixture into each of 10 flour tortillas and wrap. Place seam-side down in a baking dish. Spoon 2 tablespoons of the bacon ranch mixture into each of the remaining 10 tortillas and wrap. Place seam-side down in the baking dish.
5. Bake for 15 minutes or until brown.
6. Serve with sour cream, salsa, guacamole, etc., if desired.

There are some nights when it's a full house at the Fraser estate. Maybe Matt O'Keefe, my agent and best friend, is in town on business. Or maybe it's Jordan, the guy who does all my body work. Or maybe it's a film crew looking to get in one more shoot before I go deep into my hibernation training mode and shut everyone out. That's not to mention Tia and Shane, who are well aware where the best meal in town is. Regardless of who it is, Sammy's going to cook for them, and there will be trays of food to show for it. Even if you're laser-focused on training, a night with friends can be the perfect way to escape the pressure for a bit.

WORKOUT

10 Sets   M 100 lbs/W 70 lbs
50 GHD Sit-Ups
50 D-Ball Squats
50 D-Ball Step-Overs
50 D-Ball Squats
50 GHD Sit-Ups
50 Pull-Ups
150 Double-Unders

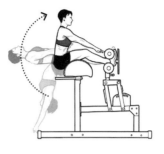

GHD Sit-Ups

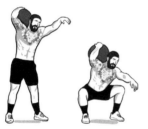

D-Ball Squats

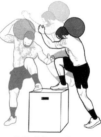

D-Ball Step-Overs

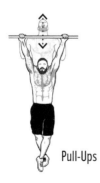

Pull-Ups

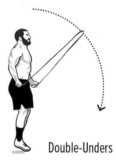

Double-Unders

WORKOUT

40–30–20 Calorie SkiErg
10–8–6 Sandbag over 48" Box

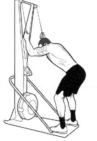
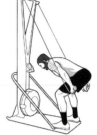

SkiErg

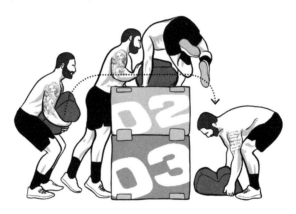

Sandbag over 48" Box

WORKOUT: *Farmer's Hold*

Accumulate *3:00* @ Body Weight

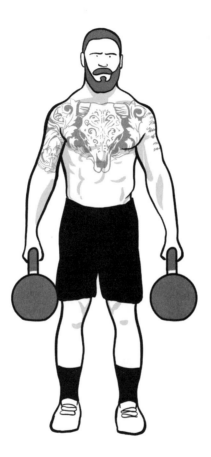

WORKOUT

100-Calorie Row
80 Wall-Balls
60 GHD Sit-Ups
40 Box Jumps
96 OH Walking Lunges

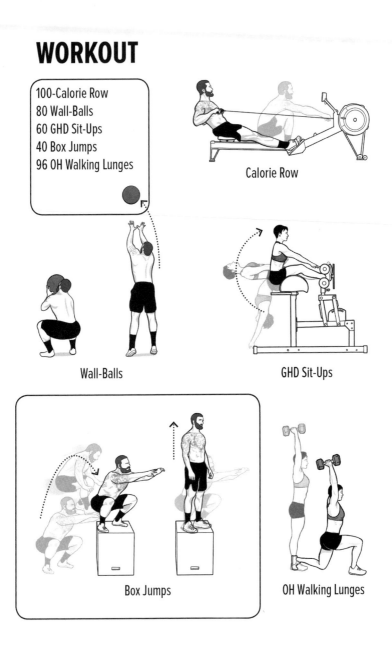

Calorie Row

Wall-Balls

GHD Sit-Ups

Box Jumps

OH Walking Lunges

EMOM for 32 mins
Minute 1: Row 22 calories
Minute 2: Bike 21 calories
Minute 3: Ski 20 calories
Minute 4: Rest

EMOM for 40 mins
18 cal row
16 cal bike

For time
800m run
3,000m row
800m run
3,000m row
800m run

2 sets
For time
27 cal ski
27 cal Echo Bike
Rest: 1 min
21 cal ski
21 cal Echo Bike
Rest: 1 min
15 cal ski
15 cal Echo Bike
Rest: 1 min
9 cal ski
9 cal Echo Bike
Rest: 5 mins between sets

3 sets
3,200m, Assault Bike (290 watts, damper 6.5)
Run 800m

4 sets
4 min AMRAP
40 cal row
25 cal bike
Max burpee
Rest: 2 mins between sets

4 sets
4 min AMRAP
40 cal row
25 cal bike
Max burpees
Rest: 2 mins between sets

C2 Bike Erg
Warm-up
60 sec @ 6K pace
30 sec @ easy
60 sec @ 4K pace
30 sec @ easy
30 sec @ 2K pace
Then
10K @ 1:47
Rest: 5 mins
8K @ 1:45
Rest: 4 mins
6K @ 1:43
Rest: 3 mins
4K @ 1:41
Rest: 2 mins
2K @ 1:39

2 sets
Start new set @ 10 min
42–30–18 row
21–15–9 Echo Bike

Workouts to Improve Your Swimming
Courtesy of Chris Hinshaw

Kick only

2 × (100 kick, long fins, 30 sec
 rest)
Rest: 1 min
50 kick at max effort, no fins,
 10 sec rest
100 recovery kick, long fins,
 30 sec rest
50 kick at max effort, no fins,
 10 sec rest
100 recovery kick, long fins,
 30 sec rest

Kick only

4 × (50 kick, short fins, 15 sec
 rest)
Rest: 1 min
50 kick at max effort, no fins,
 10 sec rest
100 recovery kick, short fins,
 30 sec rest
50 kick at max effort, no fins,
 10 sec rest
100 recovery kick, short fins,
 30 sec rest

Swim

8 × 50 on 1:10 (build to sprint
 within each 50)
5 × 100 on 2:10
Rest: 30 secs
4 × 100 on 2:00
Rest: 30 secs
3 × 100 on 2:00
Rest: 30 secs
2 × 100 on 1:50
Rest: 30 secs
1 × 100 fast (sub 1:40)
100 easy

Swim

4 × 100 swim on
 2:15, 2:00, 1:45, 1:30
100 easy swim
400 pull on 7:30
4 × 75 swim on 1:40, 1:30, 1:20,
 1:10
100 easy swim
300 pull on 5:30
4 × 50 swim on 60 sec, 55 sec,
 50 sec, 45 sec
100 easy swim
200 pull on 3:45

Workouts to Improve Your Running

3 Sets of 4 rounds
1:00 run
Rest: :30
Rest: 1:30 between sets

For time
800m run
100 push-ups
800m run
200 air squats
800m run
100 push-ups
800m run

Track
1,200m
800m
400m
400m
800m
1,200m
Rest: 3 mins between each

Workouts to Improve Your Rowing

Row

2,500m @ 1:45 pace
Rest: 6 mins
2,500m @ 1:42 pace

Row

7 sets
500m @ 1:41
100m slow
250m @ 1:38
150m slow
No rest between sets

Row

3 sets
750m @ 1:40
550m @ 1:38
350m @ 1:36
200m hard
Rest: 1 min between intervals
Rest: 3 mins between sets

5 Sets

250m hard
Rest: 30 secs

Every 2 mins for 6 sets

10 cal row
25 wall-balls

10 Sets

500m row
Rest: 1 min
(Your score is your slowest
    round)

Row

3 sets
1,500m @ 1:45
Rest: 90 secs
900m @ 1:42
Rest: 60 secs
3 rounds
200m @ 1:35
Rest: 30 secs between rounds
Rest: 4 mins between sets

3

Speed

After the heartbreak of narrowly losing the 2015 Games, I took stock of my physical weaknesses: My deadlift was barely competitive. I couldn't swim in open water. I was afraid of long sets of toes-to-bar. But there was one movement that I knew needed more work than all the others combined: my sprinting.

I took 37th out of 39 in the sprint event, and my running technique was so bad that Coach Polakowski reached out to me afterward. We'd always worked together on weightlifting, but he considered himself a track coach who used lifting as a tool and offered to let me join his track team. I was grateful for the help and agreed, not exactly realizing that I'd be running with my town's middle and high school kids.

It was before the spring season, when the Vermont winter was still too crushing to train outside, so all of us—the dozens of kids from the middle and high school—were crammed into the indoor gym. I could tell that everyone was staring at me, probably assuming that I was a new assistant coach, but when Coach Pol blew his whistle, I lined up with everyone else and did the butt kickers, high knees, and heel walks.

Over the next few months, my sprinting got better, but those improvements also made me realize that speed is about much more than stepping up and driving down. I started to look for hacks everywhere else, from how I loaded the strongman yoke to whether I did a burpee and touched the rings with the front of my hands or the back.

In that way, speed isn't just how fast you can run 100 meters or do butterfly pull-ups. It's a mindset that you have to apply to everything.

Speed Technique 101

EXERCISE: *Sprinting Technique Work*

15 sets of 40-meter sprints
for quality (not speed)

I trained with the Essex high school team two to three times a week for about four months, and it turns out that sprinting is like Olympic weightlifting in three important ways.

For one, technique is everything, and what I was doing during the suicide sprints in 2015 was totally backward. I figured that you'd want to reach your front foot out as far as possible to cover a lot of ground, right? Wrong. I also thought that you should land with your toe first so you had plenty of cushion to rebound off. Wrong again. And finally, it seemed obvious that you'd need to keep tension throughout your torso and diaphragm to give you more power. Most wrong of all.

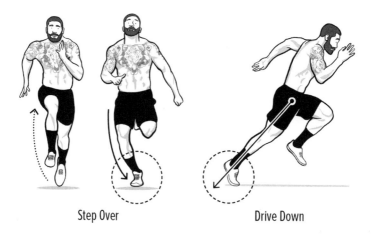

Step Over   Drive Down

In terms of your stride, the goal is to punch the ground and generate as much force as possible. To do that, when you bring your tail leg up, you want to step over the opposite knee and then drive that foot down into the ground so it lands directly underneath you with your toe pulled up toward the sky. Step over, drive down. Step over, drive down. Your stride will be shorter, but the net effect is a faster sprint. And once you've mastered the lower-body technique, you can focus on the upper body.

Just like with Olympic lifting, it's best to relax under tension. Imagine trying to snatch with your triceps flexed the entire time. It'd be impossible, and the same thing is true for sprinting. The more you tense your arms and scrunch your face and try to go

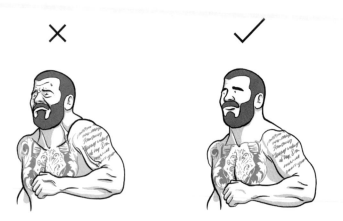

faster, the slower you'll end up. To make sure you aren't running with your elbows out wide or your shoulders hunched into your ears, set up a camera and film yourself.

WORKOUT: *Box Jump Speed Work*

3 sets of 10 (M 30"/W 24")
Rest: *00:40* between sets

The last similarity between sprinting and Olympic lifting is that you improve in the warm-ups, activations, and drills more than when you're trying to beat your personal best. During Coach Pol's track workouts, the sprinting itself was surprisingly short, no more than 40 meters and with three minutes of rest between sets. That meant that the majority of the time was practicing the step-over, drive down, and activating our fast-twitch muscles through jumping: vertical jumps, broad jumps, quick rebounds, and jumping off our heels and toes. Then we'd work on starts, which is something that I'd never thought to do.

Gradually, I felt my technique getting better but had no idea if I was faster. Coach Pol always paired me with the kid who would become a Vermont state champion in the 100, and he would blow my doors off every race. This is what I needed. I train best when I feel scared that my hard work won't pay off because then I feel like I have to focus on every little detail to get progress wherever I can.

So even though it was humbling being an adult professional athlete training with kids (and losing), I liked track practice, especially the pace of it. Unlike the rest of my training, these workouts didn't hurt from start to finish. I was never on the verge of blacking out or wondering where I could squeak out more rest. So I was a little bummed when I had to start working on the other weaknesses in my tool chest. Coach Pol said I could drop in anytime I wanted and even gave me a set of starting blocks so I could keep practicing on my own.

WORKOUT: *Shuttle Run Drill*

3 attempts: record your fastest time

Coach Pol did an amazing job, but he was just one of the many experts I reached out to for help with running. Hinshaw was another, and a third was Matt Hewett, the head of strength and conditioning at Tennessee Tech and a big competitive CrossFit athlete. Polakowski had taught me to sprint, but not how to decelerate, turn, and accelerate again, which is what the sprinting at the Games usually looks like.

By the time I linked up with Hewett, in 2017, Sammy and I had moved to Cookeville. At this point, there was no doubt that CrossFit was now my full-time job, so I was reaching out to anyone who could potentially help me. Hewett was a great resource.

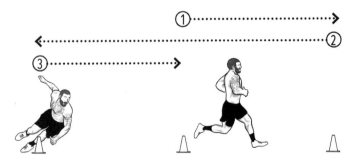

At the Games, sprinting is typically paired with another movement, like a sled push or a set of obstacles, so Hewett worked with me to better position my body to change directions. One of the drills we practiced was the 5–10–5 shuttle run drill, which they also use at the NFL Combine. To do it, set up three cones that are each 5 yards apart. When the timer starts, dash to the left and touch the cone, sprint 10 yards and touch the cone on the far side, then sprint back to the middle. If you can get under four seconds, you should consider quitting CrossFit to pursue football.

WORKOUT: *Hinshaw's Sprint Intervals*

16 Rounds
200 meters in *00:38*, followed by
100 meters at whatever pace is needed to
keep the 200 meters at *00:38* or below

After I worked with Polakowski and Hewett, my stride looked and felt better, but it took me much longer to understand how to pace. Just like with lifting, I never wanted to throttle back on my sprints. It was go, go, go as fast as possible for as long as possible, until one day when it clicked with Hinshaw.

We were up in Vermont in the middle of summer, and working out in the heat is already miserable for me. I'm almost always warm, which is why our house stays at 67 degrees and why I end a big workout with my head in the watercooler. People think it's funny when they see it, but especially during the Games, when we're on AstroTurf that's baked in the sun all day, my internal temperature can rise so high that I'm on the verge of passing out.

But there was no time to dunk my head during this workout. During the 20 minutes, I wouldn't even have time to drink water—or catch my breath.

I didn't realize when we started that Hinshaw had designed this workout specifically to teach me a lesson, so I approached it how I always did. He said that my 200 was supposed to be 38 seconds, so I was going to do it in 37 because faster was better. I did that for the first five rounds, and my 100-meter times started shooting up: 40 seconds, then 42 and 45. I was killing myself to make those 200s in 37 seconds and refused to relent. Faster was better.

Around the 8th or 9th round, Hinshaw hopped onto the track and told me I had to hold back on the 200s. I didn't want to, but I was so hot I was dizzy. Plus, if my 100s got any slower, I knew I'd miss the point of the workout. So I dropped the pace on the 200 ever so slightly, and the 100s started to creep back down to 38 seconds.

This experience taught me a lesson I've used ever since: One second matters. If you throttle back just a bit, it can make the difference between redlining and sustaining your pace, but it's a skill you have to practice.

WORKOUT: *Nasty Nancy*

> **5 Rounds**
> Run 500 meters
> 15 Overhead Squats
> 15 Bar-Facing Burpees
> M 185 lbs/W 125 lbs
> **My time:** *17:50*

If you already do CrossFit, you probably hate when running comes up in a workout. You shouldn't. Especially during a workout with more challenging movements, it gives you flexibility to adjust your pace and recover.

In this workout, from Phase One of the 2020 Games, the real work is the overhead squats and the bar-facing burpees, so I want you to try this workout twice. The first time, record your splits on the run. Did you come out of the gate too hot and then implode by the fourth round? Did you start slow and gradually get faster? Did you hold a pretty consistent pace throughout?

For the second attempt, use your average score from the first attempt and add five seconds. That's your new pace. It's going to feel like you're practically standing still, especially if there are other athletes passing you by, but I want you to see how a relatively small amount of recovery can have a huge effect. Ultimately, maintaining a consistent speed is better than sprinting the 500 meters, doing two overhead squats, then spending half a minute with your hands on your knees. Learning how to properly pace is fundamental to CrossFit—and something that still makes me nervous.

WORKOUT: *Mary*

AMRAP in 20
5 Handstand Push-Ups
10 Pistols (alternating legs)
15 Pull-Ups

I was scared when "Mary" came up at the 2019 Games. For starters, the coliseum that night was unusually hot, and with 15 dudes on the floor and no fans to move the air, I was pretty sure I'd overheat if I didn't hold myself back for at least the first 10 minutes. However, I didn't have much of a buffer. I was in the lead by just two points, and Noah Ohlsen, the guy in second, was definitely capable of winning the workout.

When it came to strategy, though, I had a problem: I hate AMRAPs, especially for an event this long. How can I be sure that my pace is the right pace? It's not like one strategy makes the workout easy and pain-free. They're all going to hurt, so what's the perfect mix of discomfort and recovery to get the highest score?

I don't know. Unless you're on an Assault Bike, rower, or Ski-Erg, where you can see the wattage, strokes per minute, and calories the entire time, it's almost impossible to be sure.

That's why Hinshaw trained me in 13 different time domains: 180 minutes, 120 minutes, 90, 60, 40, 20, 10, 5, 3, 2, 1, thirty seconds, and ten seconds. In any workout, the cardio portion is going to fall somewhere near one of these categories, and I know from muscle memory about how fast I should go.

At the 2019 Games, the strategy I chose paid off. I didn't overheat and ended up getting second in Mary, just a few reps shy of Ohlsen.

Thankfully, AMRAPs don't come up often at the Games, but neither does my favorite kind of workout: every minute on the minute (EMOM). These are great because you're told how much work to do and how long to do it in, so there's no holding back. If you fail, you fail, and the workout's over, so you can really push into a dark place.

For that reason I recommend trying Mary twice. The first time, do it as an AMRAP. The second time, choose a slightly higher score, divide it by 20, and now you've got an EMOM. You may do even better when you don't have to worry about your pacing and can save your mental energy.

WORKOUT: *Aeneas*

3 Rounds
10 Thrusters (M 85 lbs/W 55 lbs)
33-foot Yoke Carry, add weight
33-foot Yoke Carry, add weight
33-foot Yoke Carry
M 85-pound Thruster, 425–565–665-pound Yoke Carries
W 55-pound Thruster, 345–405–445-pound Yoke Carries
My time: *3:56*

Now that we've covered some of the technical aspects of speed, I want to talk about my speed mentality. This event looks like it's all about strength and endurance, but remember: Everything at the Games is about speed.

In 2015, I wouldn't have thought twice about how I loaded the yoke here. I would've just grabbed the plates, thrown them on, and been angry and surprised if they hit an edge and rolled away. But by 2018, I'd become a different athlete. Not only did I want to do everything possible to avoid a mistake, even if it was one in a hundred, but I'd also learned that the time it takes to load a yoke is just as valuable as the time it takes to do your reps, so why would I leave any part of the workout to chance? Why wouldn't I practice picking up plates if I practice thrusters, which take just as long?

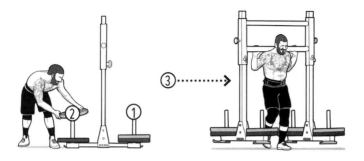

When it comes to loading the yoke, placement is everything. If you load the back plates first, you end up at the front of the yoke and need to move to the back to pick it up. If you do it the opposite way, you can just lift and go.

Did my loading strategy make the difference in this workout? No, but two seconds is two seconds regardless of how they're spent. So remember: Once the timer starts, every movement you make is part of your score.

WORKOUT: *Ringer 2*

15–10–5 Reps for time
Burpees
Overhead Squats (M 135 lbs/W 95 lbs)
Time cap: *5:00*
My time: *3:06*

The shorter the event, the more you have to look for advantages, and everybody knew that this event from the 2019 Games was going to be a barn burner. I mean, half the people sitting in the stands could have done it without stopping, so I had to be fast and cut time wherever possible. Besides making sure I grabbed the bar and got going, I couldn't do a lot when it came to the overhead squats, so I analyzed the burpees.

In terms of pacing, I knew that I do burpees between two and three seconds: three if I want to recover, two if I'm looking to move quick. There was no question there about which speed to choose, but could I make the movement itself even faster? Unlike a normal burpee, in this workout we had to touch a set of rings at the top of our jump. All the rings were set at the same height, so some of the taller guys would already have an advantage. I'd have to jump about a foot and couldn't waste any extra energy.

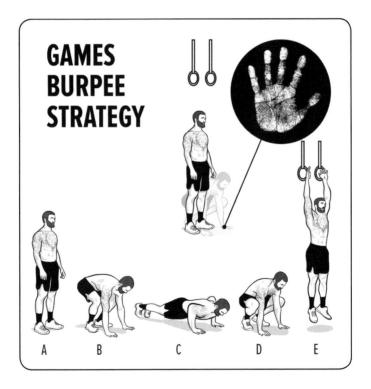

GAMES
BURPEE
STRATEGY

A   B   C   D   E

I came up with two strategies. First, I chalked up so much that I left clear handprints on the mat so I'd know exactly where to position my body to be directly underneath the rig. Then I asked the judge if I could touch the rings with the back of my hands, not the front. Using these two strategies, I barely had to look up at the top of my burpee, which is slower, takes more energy, and makes it more difficult to breathe. I also dropped into the bottom of the burpee more aggressively than I would have in the gym because we were on top of a Dollamur mat, not a hard rubber floor.

Again, is that what made the difference in that workout? Probably not. But at this point I was trailing Noah Ohlsen on the leaderboard and couldn't afford to waste even a half second. Still, going for these shortcuts was a risk. I ended up getting no-repped on my first burpee in the second round, and my penalty was even more severe on another event from the 2019 Games.

Advanced Speed Mindset Techniques

WORKOUT: *Ruck Run*

5-kilometer ruck run

Going into the 2019 Games, I was almost positive there would be a ruck run. GORUCK had been announced as a sponsor, so to train I went out and bought one of their Ruck backpacks and began to practice the best technique for adding and removing the weight.

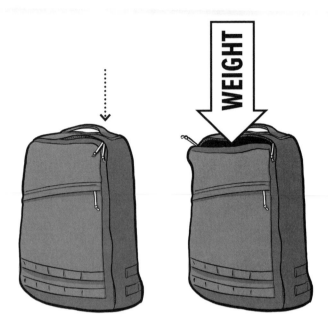

What I came up with in practice was this: Because the bag was square, I left both zippers in the top right corner. They were touching, so the bag was closed, and after I finished each lap and had to add more weight, I could throw the sack over my right shoulder, pull the top zipper to the left, grab a sandbag, throw it in, zip it back up, and toss it over my shoulder. I wasn't fumbling with grabbing the wrong zipper or looking for it down the edges of the sack. Just unzip, throw in the weight, and go.

But the sacks were designed to hold weighted plates, which fit in their own compartments like a laptop sleeve, and we were using sandbags. So during the actual event, they jostled around as we ran, and the zippers slowly came down throughout the run. Some guys had all their weight fall out at once, which was actually better because it was so noticeable that they'd stop, scoop them up, and keep running. But when my pack unzipped, only one of the 10-pound weights came out. I thought I felt something hit my foot and turned around to check, but didn't see a sandbag and was almost done with the race anyway, so I kept going.

They ended up penalizing me a full minute, the 28 seconds I was running without the sandbag, doubled and rounded up to a minute. I didn't think it was a fair penalty, but it didn't matter how I felt. That was the reality.

Still, even though it didn't pay off, I don't regret taking that calculated risk. It's better to overthink your strategy than to leave something to chance. And that's the case even for something as seemingly straightforward as an all-out sprint.

WORKOUT   1,000-meter row

The 1,000-meter row is going to feel awful no matter how you approach it, but if you want the best time, approach it as three different sections: a 300, a 400, a 300. The first 300 should be two seconds faster than your overall pace, the 400 should be two seconds slower, and the last part should be an all-out sprint.

So when I did it most recently, during Phase One of the 2020 Games, I wanted to hit a 2:58, which would average out to a 1:29 pace for both of the 500-meter splits. But I didn't pull at that speed the entire time. Instead, I rowed at a 1:27 for the first 300 meters,

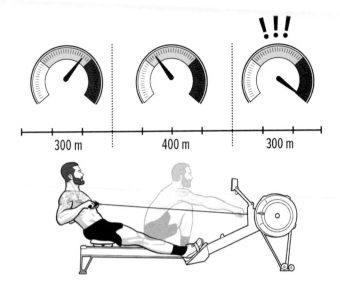

1:31 for the next 400 meters, then dropped the hammer and pulled with everything I had left, which wasn't much at that point. Still, it was better than the strategy I had when I first tried it, which was to blow myself up in the first half of the race and have nothing left in the tank for that last interval.

This time around, it worked. I ended up with 2:55.20, a new PR and good enough for 8th place. Not being among the best (or tallest) rowers in the field, I was especially happy that my strategy paid off.

But what do you do when everything you planned for goes down the drain?

WORKOUT: *14 × 14*

Row 14 sets of 250 meters at the
same pace for each interval.
Keep track of your own time.

Your speed mindset only works if you can continue making good decisions once your heart rate's jacked up. This isn't easy, but like everything else, it's a skill you can improve at. I don't listen to music or train with other people when I practice my sprint intervals, which forces me to focus on my technique, breathing, and times tables.

Let's say I need to do 16 sets of 100-meter sprints and end up with an overall average of 21 seconds for each. I keep track of my own times by acting like I'm a card-counter. I run the first 100 in 20 seconds, so I'm one point up. The next one is 22 seconds, so now I'm back to even. The third is 20 seconds again, so I'm up a point again, and so on.

On top of that, I'm also keeping track of the time when I need to start the next interval, and I'm going through the squares in my head: two times two, three times three, four times four, and on. By the end of the workout, I'm really struggling to remember my time, keep track of the "count," and calculate 14 times 14.

If you've never tried to incorporate this kind of mental training into your routine, start small. You might want to do, say, a 250-meter row every 59 seconds for 10 sets. The timing will be easy to keep track of at first and slowly get more difficult. Then you can add in other challenges, like naming state capitals or words that start with the letter Y. The better you're able to concentrate under fatigue, the fewer bozo mistakes you'll make.

WORKOUT: *Double DT*

10 Rounds for time
12 Deadlifts (M 155 lbs/W 105 lbs)
9 Hang Power Cleans (M 155 lbs/W 105 lbs)
6 Push Jerks (M 155 lbs/W 105 lbs)
My time: *11:41*

Double DT is an especially brutal workout because your back, shoulders, and grip are totally fried by the end, not to mention that your central nervous system is screaming and you can barely breathe. It's easy to make a simple mistake in that state, which I was close to doing at the Games in 2016.

Competitions aren't like normal training for a lot of reasons. Some of them are obvious: They're louder, more crowded, and higher-stake than practice. But there are subtle differences that have an impact, too, like how you have to move along the floor in a certain way. For example, during Double DT, there were 10 markers spaced out along the floor, one for every round, and you had to push the barbell forward as you completed each one. That way, the crowd could instantly see where you were in relation to the other competitors.

I don't know a lot of athletes who practice DT this way, so it's easy to forget in the heat of the moment. I was on the verge of finishing the push jerks and immediately starting the deadlifts without rolling it to the next marker. That would've been a needless, foolish mistake because I'd have to drop the barbell and waste a rep. If you make a silly mistake like that on half of the 15 events, they add up.

So when you try Double DT on your own, add something simple that you have to do between each movement, like tapping your head or saying the name of your gym. You'll be shocked how quickly you forget, so do it with a friend who can keep you accountable.

If you're hoping to compete in the sport, you need to be so well trained mentally that you don't get rattled by minor adjustments. In fact, you should be so dialed in that you spot loopholes in the rules.

WORKOUT: *2018 CrossFit Regionals Event 5*

50 Handstand Push-Ups

50 Toes-to-Bars

50-calorie Assault Bike

50 Dumbbell Box Step-Overs (M 24″/W 20″)

50-foot Right-Arm Dumbbell Overhead Lunge
(M 70 lbs/W 50 lbs)

50-foot Left-Arm Dumbbell Overhead Lunge
(M 70 lbs/W 50 lbs)

My time: *14:36*

This was a grueling chipper, and the Assault Bike, lunges, and box step-overs definitely didn't favor the shorter guys in the field. Before the event, when I was formulating my strategy, I knew there was nothing I could do to hack those first two movements (other than grow three inches in height), but what about the step-overs?

Most guys stood as close to the box as they could and did a 140-pound lunge up to the box. But if you watch me, I started four feet away and almost ran toward it while swinging the dumbbells, which helped pull me over the box. It took a bit longer, but if I tried to do this movement strict, like the guys around me, I'd have to start the step-over with my knee basically in my chin. So I was willing to sacrifice some time in the short term to be faster overall.

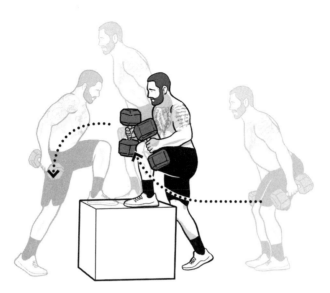

Now, I wouldn't have tried this if the step-overs were the end of the workout. But afterward we still had the lunges, and the two guys in front of me, who did the strict approach, were so winded that they literally sat down on their box for 30, maybe 40 seconds. Meanwhile, I was able to finish the step-overs, toss my box out of the way, pick up the dumbbells and start lunging.

Experiment with different step-over methods when you try this workout, and you might find that what's quickest for any single movement isn't necessarily the best for your overall strategy.

WORKOUT: *2223 Intervals*

> *2:00* On, *1:00* Off
> 2 Rope Climbs
> 10/7-calorie SkiErg
> Max Overhead Squat
> 4th round extended to 3 minutes
> Go until 75 reps of Overhead Squat are complete
> M 155 lbs/W 105 lbs
> **My time:** *10:54*

This event came at the end of the 2017 Games, and I needed any advantage I could get. No one knew that I'd torn the LCL in my knee a few days earlier. I'd made sure to hide the injury from everyone, even Sammy and O'Keefe, so I wouldn't freak myself out or let the other athletes know they had a competitive edge. But after 11 events, I was hurting.

Just like with Double DT, you had to move the barbell across the floor as you progressed through the overhead squats. The first 30 reps were broken up into sets of 10, and after that it was 15 sets of three, each with its own designated box. Between the boxes, you could do whatever you wanted. You could keep the barbell overhead, bring it down to your shoulders, dump it and push it forward, whatever. Still, that was a ton of space to cover, and I wanted to minimize my transitions as much as possible.

While most of the other guys squatted in the center of the box, I went to the very front, so my toes were just about touching the

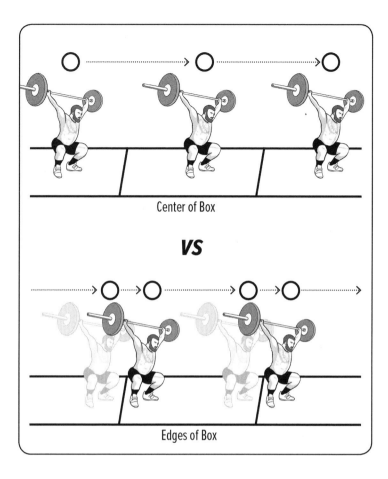

Center of Box

VS

Edges of Box

line. I'd do my three squats there, take one step into the next box, and do three more. Then I'd drop the bar to my shoulders and walk to the very front of the next section. That way, I was basically doing sets of six instead of three.

This hack was especially helpful with so many overhead squats to do in such a small window of time. In fact, I noticed that a few other guys did the same thing, which is another component of the speed mindset: Strategy doesn't just mean focusing on what you're doing. You also have to be aware of where your competitors are, too.

WORKOUT: *Second Cut*

Row 800 meters
66 Kettlebell Jerks (M 16 kg/W 12 kg)
132-foot Handstand Walk
Time cap: *10:00*

Instead of running through multiplication tables during competition, I shift that focus to the guys around me. During an event like the one-rep snatch, it's fairly easy to understand what's going on because the action is controlled. Even though there's a lot to remember—not just the heaviest lift from the earlier heats, but also what the 14 guys around me are attempting—my heart rate isn't jacked up, and after so many years of lifting I know the weight of a barbell just from looking at it.

It gets a little more challenging during a workout where we're all moving at once, especially for something as chaotic as the second event at the 2019 Games. There were 36 other guys in my heat, and we all started on rowers lined up next to one another. It was impossible to see the screen of a guy on the other side of the field, but I could listen to the announcers, who always track the front-runners throughout the event.

In fact, I listen to them and the judges next to me more than I listen to my own judge—not that I can hear them well to begin with. My hearing hasn't improved since I was a kid, and one of my biggest concerns during competition is that I'll get no-repped, not realize it, then have to do the movement all over again. So the first thing I tell my judge is to yell any no-reps as loudly as possible.

I wasn't the first off the rower for that event, but from listening to the announcers, I knew I wasn't that far behind the leaders. Like I said in the strength chapter, I noticed that everyone else was doing proper jerks with the kettlebells, so I decided to do push presses and cranked through 44 of the 66 reps. Then I put down the bells and looked around. I wasn't in the lead yet, so instead of taking the breather I wanted, I finished the presses, shook out my arms, and got ready to handstand-walk.

Even though I'm pretty comfortable on my hands, each section of the handstand walk was 44 feet, and you had to go back to the start if you didn't make it all the way through. But in my peripheral vision I saw a few guys who were right behind me, so I finished the entire 132 feet more or less in one shot.

In this case, I was able to hold on and finish with a faster time than I would've gotten if I'd done the workout on my own. But part of the speed mindset is also knowing when it's best to sacrifice a good score in order to gain the psychological edge.

WORKOUT: *First Cut*

4 Rounds
Run 400 meters
3 Legless Rope Climbs
7 Squat Snatches (M 185 lbs/W 130 lbs)
Time cap: *20:00*
My time: *15:07*

If you're aiming to be an elite competitor, the ideal strategy isn't necessarily the one that allows you to do the workout fastest.

Going into the 2019 Games, Pat Vellner was telling everyone he could that he was going to beat me. He'd taken second the year before and was looking to make a statement during this first workout, so I knew that, of the 46 other guys in our heat, Vellner was the one to watch. And there he was, in the lane right next to me on the AstroTurf.

For the first half of the event, Vellner and I were side by side as we ran off the field, around a blind corner, and outside the stadium. Gradually the other athletes started to thin out, and he and I were leading the pack by the end of the second round. And that's when I sabotaged my score.

I'd normally throttle back in this situation. Vellner and I were alone on the run, and we weren't in the final round yet. We weren't racing. But I knew that the commentary for the rest of the week was going to be based off this first workout, and I wanted to make a statement of my own. So I decided to break the rubber band.

I set off at a reasonable pace as I left the AstroTurf, and when I got to that blind corner just before the stadium exit, I went for a full sprint. I was so fatigued that I'm sure it didn't look like I was running any faster, but I disappeared to Vellner. In an interview after the event, he said he thought he was close when we left the stadium, but I was long gone the next time he saw me. My strategy worked, and he never knew that I blew myself up in the process and was struggling to get through that fourth round.

Though I recovered better than Vellner, who missed a few reps of the 185-pound snatches and ended up in 9th place, it wasn't by much. I'm 100 percent certain that I could have done that workout with a faster overall time if I had paced it more appropriately, but Vellner and I were trying to break each other, and establishing that upper hand early was worth the risk of bombing out.

Don't take this as permission to lead with your ego. If you're more concerned about establishing dominance than setting and holding the right pace, you're going to lose 99 times out of 100. But if you train with the humility of a grown man practicing sprinting technique with the high school track team, you may find yourself in a situation where you have two choices. You can pray that you don't get passed by the athlete behind you, or you can hit the blind turn, start sprinting, and hope you break the rubber band.

The Speed Mentality

JOURNAL ENTRY—Where in the workout are you giving up your competitive advantage? Is it beforehand, when you're nervously pacing? Is it during, when you can't help but groan during every rep? Is it afterward, when you collapse to the floor and convulse in a puddle of your own sweat?

Unless I am fully blacked out or on the verge of overheating and passing out, I don't lie down after I finish a workout, especially a sprint barn burner like Ringer 1 or Ringer 2 at the 2019 Games. I wanted to then, but I knew it wasn't the smart choice. Pacing back and forth would help flush the lactic acid out of my body, but even more important, I needed the other dudes to know that I wasn't fading. Instead, they'd be smarter to focus on not getting caught by the guys behind them. Even after you cross that finish line, the Rubber Band Effect is always in play.

I'm not saying you have to be a robot every second. I'm not. From my first competition in 2012 to my last one in 2020, I was nervous before every event. Not like oh, a little bit of adrenaline and butterflies in the stomach. Like, dry heaving or outright puking while I was in the athlete corral before our heat was called. Something like that is pretty difficult to hide, so I always made up for it as soon as I walked onto the floor. The nerves, doubt, and fear all disappeared, and I was ready to blackout in the workout before I showed any weakness.

So identify where you show the most vulnerability and how important it is to you. For example, I learned I could resist collapsing to the ground after a workout if I knew I'd get to dunk my head in the cooler a few seconds later. Pinpointing where the pain feels most intense will help you build a strategy around it.

Eating for Speed—Slimming Down

Body mass is great when you're looking to get stronger, but it makes a lot of other movements more difficult, whether it's sprinting, doing massive sets of toes-to-bar without your grip giving out, or straining from the bottom of a six-inch deficit handstand push-up. That's the tricky part about CrossFit. You've got to be able to do it all on the same day—a one-rep max deadlift and a sled push down the field and back.

I preferred to compete on the lighter side, which was one of the most difficult changes to make after the 2015 Games. I knew that I had to fully commit if I wanted to keep pursuing CrossFit, and that would mean eating lighter meals that allowed me to slim down when I needed to.

Sweet & Simple Chicken Salad

1 rotisserie chicken, with skin removed, chopped

1 cup red grapes, halved

$1/4$ cup walnuts, chopped

$1/4$ cup mayonnaise

Salad greens, wrap, or toasted bread for serving (optional)

1. Add the chicken, grapes, walnuts, and mayonnaise to a large mixing bowl. Toss until well combined.
2. Chill in the refrigerator.
3. Serve the chicken salad over a bed of greens, in a wrap, or on toasted bread for a sandwich , if desired.

For the first few years of CrossFit, I was a college student eating fried food off the trucks behind the library. Even though I knew it made me feel like trash, I didn't care. I didn't have the time, money, or skills to improve my diet, and maybe that's where you are now. You don't have a sponsorship from a meal delivery service or a partner who loves to cook. I understand. But there's no denying that what you fuel your body with shapes the kind of athlete you become. So start slow if you have to, like making sure you have a Tupperware of chicken salad in the fridge that you can throw into your bag in the morning.

Grilled Mexican Street Corn

4 ears of corn, halved

2 tablespoons olive oil

1 tablespoon kosher salt

1 tablespoon chipotle mayo

3 tablespoon cotija cheese, shredded

Cilantro for garnish

1. Set the grill to medium-high heat.
2. Drizzle the ears of corn with the olive oil and sprinkle with the salt. Place the corn on the grill for 20 to 25 minutes, turning frequently every 3 to 5 minutes to evenly char the corn.
3. Remove the corn from the grill and smother in the chipotle mayo. Sprinkle with the cotija cheese and cilantro and serve.

When I decided I was going to make a real play for the 2016 Games, I was around 205 pounds, probably the heaviest I've ever been as a CrossFit athlete. But I told myself that I'd do everything possible in the next ten months to become a champion, starting with my diet. You don't have to be this extreme. Like I said in Chapter 1, it's the 1 percent of the .01 percent of athletes who have even a chance of becoming competitive CrossFit athletes and staying so obsessively focused on your diet definitely messes with your head. After the season, I'd end up bingeing on cookies and cheesecake to make up for all the moments I couldn't eat what I wanted.

Harvest Quinoa Salad

2 cups butternut squash, cubed

1 cup delicata squash, sliced

1 tablespoon olive oil

Salt and pepper

1 cup cooked quinoa

3 cups baby spinach

$^1/_2$ cup shelled edamame

$^1/_4$ cup dried blueberries

$^1/_4$ cup roasted hazelnuts, chopped

$^1/_2$ cup plain Greek yogurt

1 tablespoon lemon juice

2 tablespoons apple cider vinegar

2 teaspoons garlic, minced

2 teaspoons Dijon mustard

1. Preheat the oven to 425°F.
2. On a large rimmed baking sheet, toss the butternut squash and delicata squash with the olive oil and salt and pepper to taste. Roast in the oven for 25 minutes. Toss and return to the oven to roast for an additional 20 minutes until golden. Remove the roasted squash from the oven and allow to cool for 10 minutes.
3. In a large bowl, toss the quinoa, spinach, edamame, dried blueberries, and roasted hazelnuts. Add the cooled roasted squash. Toss to combine.
4. In a small bowl, whisk the yogurt, lemon juice, apple cider vinegar, garlic, Dijon, and a pinch of pepper.

5. Dress the salad with 3 to 4 tablespoons of the yogurt dressing. Store the remaining dressing in a mason jar in the fridge for future use.

By the 2017 Games, Sammy realized that it was best to phase out gluten and dairy from my diet. I'm not lactose intolerant and don't have celiac disease, but eating both gives me a bit of inflammation, nothing that the average person would notice but enough to potentially make a difference in my recovery. However, most of the time I wouldn't even realize that she'd cut them out. I didn't do the shopping for our house, and Sammy would make the change without telling me. She'd switch to gluten-free bread or replace the cheese in my sandwich with an extra slice of avocado, and I was usually too exhausted or distracted by training to know what I was missing. This was a huge lifeline during the most intense parts of my training, when I already felt deprived of most things.

Dan Dan Ramen

1 pound ground pork

2 teaspoons hoisin sauce

1 teaspoon white wine

1 teaspoon dark soy sauce

$1/2$ teaspoon five-spice powder

4 ramen cakes, seasoning pack discarded

1 tablespoon olive oil

1 pint shiitake mushrooms, sliced

1 tablespoon fresh ginger, grated

2 tablespoons shallots, minced

Sauce

3 tablespoons soy sauce

2 tablespoons sesame paste (2 tablespoons tahini plus
2 teaspoons sesame oil)

1 tablespoon white wine

2 teaspoons dark soy sauce

$1/4$ teaspoon five-spice powder

$1/4$ cup chili oil crunch

$1/4$ cup reserved water from the noodles

1. In a large skillet over medium-high heat, cook the ground pork. When little pink remains, add the hoisin sauce, white wine, dark soy sauce, and five-spice powder. Stir to combine and cook an additional 2 to 4 minutes until fully cooked. Remove the meat from the pan.

2. Bring a pot of water to a boil over high heat and cook the ramen according to the package instructions (without the seasoning packet). Strain the water and reserve $1/4$ cup for the sauce. Set the noodles aside.

3. To the skillet where the pork was cooked, add the olive oil. Cook the shiitake mushrooms over medium-high heat about 5 minutes until lightly browned. Add the ginger and shallots and cook until fragrant, about 2 minutes.

4. Meanwhile, make the sauce. In a small bowl, whisk together the soy sauce, sesame paste, white wine, dark soy sauce, five-spice powder, chili oil crunch, and reserved water. Add the sauce to the mushrooms and cook on low heat for 2 minutes.

5. Remove from the heat. Add the noodles to the skillet. Top with the meat and scallions and toss to combine. Serve.

If you're also considering cutting something out from your diet, I encourage you to do it for the right reasons. Don't just do it because that's what Mat Fraser does, or because you read it on a blog somewhere. It's easy to get caught up in diet trends, especially when they're taking over your social media, but what I hope you take away from this manual is that you have to listen to your body. I could tell that I had a little extra inflammation because I spent all day checking in with myself, so I knew exactly how I should feel if I slept nine hours, had two espressos in the morning, ate a moderate-sized lunch, and was pulling a 1:40 split on the rower for my final 500. You probably won't get that same level of body awareness, but start to notice how your diet affects how you feel physically and emotionally. Then you can make decisions from there. Also: I didn't eliminate dairy and gluten from my diet year-round, just at the height of competition season, when I was using every tool I had to fully recover.

Red Beans and Rice

1 pound Cajun smoked chicken sausage, sliced

1 tablespoon olive oil

1 onion, chopped

1 orange bell pepper, chopped

2 cloves garlic, minced

2 (15-ounce) cans red beans, drained and rinsed

1 tablespoon Creole seasoning

$2^{1}/_{2}$ cups vegetable broth

2 cups cooked white rice

$^{1}/_{4}$ cup scallions, sliced

1. In a large skillet over medium heat, cook the chicken sausage until browned. Remove from the pan and set aside on a plate.
2. In the same skillet, heat the olive oil. When the oil shimmers, add the chopped onion and pepper and cook for 5 to 7 minutes. Add the garlic and cook for an additional 1 to 2 minutes until translucent. Return the chicken sausage to the skillet.
3. Add the beans and seasoning and cook for 3 to 5 minutes.
4. Add the broth and simmer for 5 to 10 minutes.
5. Mix in the cooked white rice and simmer for an additional 3 to 5 minutes.
6. Serve topped with sliced scallions. Enjoy!

In addition to cooking all the meals, Sammy also became a master in distracting me. There'd be times that I'd request something that she knew I shouldn't eat, like a vat of mac and cheese. Instead of making that for me, she'd come up with something that was equally delicious but a little less dense, and it'd make me forget all about a giant bowl of fat and carbs. Being able to still have some variety in my diet was a great way to stay focused.

Additional Speed Training

WORKOUT

> **3 Sets**
> *1:00* Bike
> 3/3 Overhead Squats (5 sec tempo)
> *:20* L-Sit Hold on Parallette

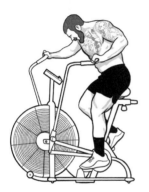

Bike

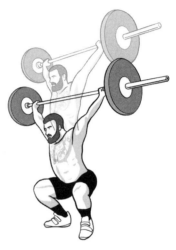

Overhead Squat

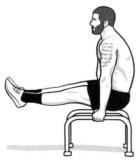

L-Sit on Parallette

WORKOUT

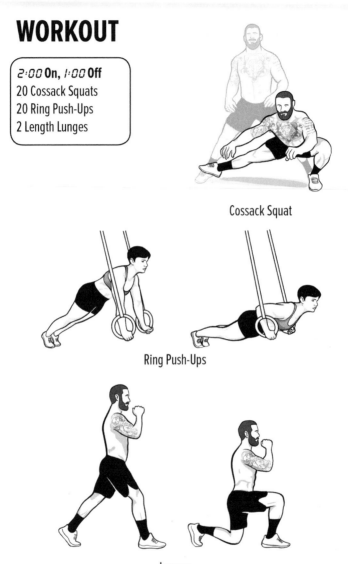

2:00 **On,** 1:00 **Off**
20 Cossack Squats
20 Ring Push-Ups
2 Length Lunges

Cossack Squat

Ring Push-Ups

Lunges

WORKOUT

2:00 **On,** *1:00* **Off**
30-Calorie SkiErg
5 Bar Muscle-Ups
2 Sandbag Cleans (M 200 lbs/W 150 lbs)
Max Burpees
Accumulate 50 Burpees

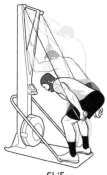

SkiErg

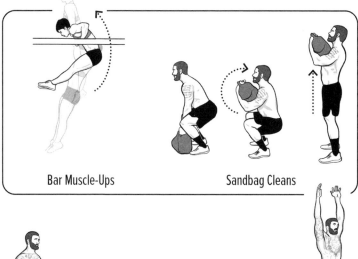

Bar Muscle-Ups   Sandbag Cleans

Burpees

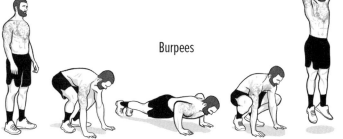

WORKOUT

EMOM for *40:00*
Min 1: 15-Calorie Echo Bike
Min 2: 5 D-Ball (M 150 lbs/W100 lbs)
Min 3: 15-Calorie Row
Min 4: 10 Dumbbell Snatches (M 70 lbs/W 50 lbs)

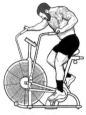

Echo Bike

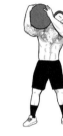

D-Ball

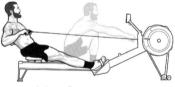

Calorie Row

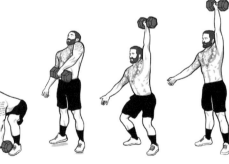

Dumbbell Snatches

EMOM for 10 mins

Min 1: 15m handstand walk

Min 2: 35 sec hollow hold

EMOM for 18 mins

Minute 1: 18 GHD

Minute 2: 18 chest-to-bar
pull-ups

Minute 3: 18 box jumps
(M 24"/W 20")

EMOM for 14 mins

Minute 1: 8 strict ring dips

Minute 2: 6 shoulder-to-overhead
heavy dumbbell

EMOM for 10 mins

16 wall-balls

WORKOUT

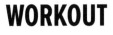

15:00 **AMRAP** with vest
25 Push-Ups
35 Air Squats
50 Step-Ups

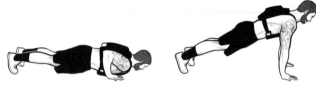

Push-Ups

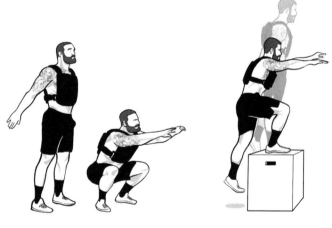

Air Squats   Step-Ups

WORKOUT

/0:00 AMRAP
Alternating single arm Devil's Press (M 50 lbs/W 35 lbs)

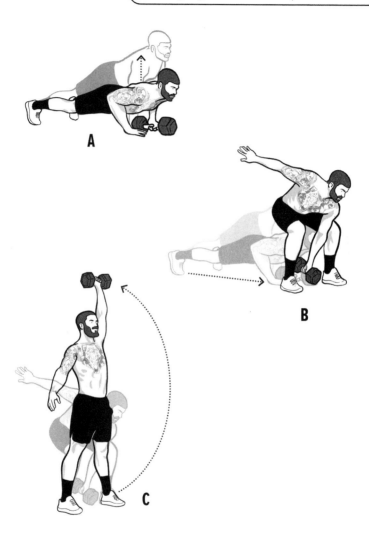

A

B

C

3 Sets

5 min AMRAP

9 power cleans (medium-light)

15 lateral burpees

21 cal Assault Bike

Rest: 5 mins between sets

10 min AMRAP

16 pull-ups

16 alternating goblet box step-
ups (heavy)

16 toes-to-bars

16 thrusters (medium)

10 min AMRAP

Alternating single-arm devil's
press (heavy)

15 min AMRAP (with vest)

25 push-ups

35 air squats

50 step-ups

My Six-Week Speed Program Before the 2020 Games, Courtesy of Matt Hewett

Track Workouts

Track Warm-Up

400m

300m

2 × 200m

AirRunner

3 sets

400m 1350

Rest: 1 min

800m 1250

Rest: 2 mins

1,200m 1150

Rest: 4 mins

Hill Sprints

7 sets

:36 up

1:00 down

Rest: :20

4 sets

300m (18–19 secs/100m)

Rest: :90

600m sub 2 mins

400m slow

200m (18–19 secs/100m)

Rest: 3 mins between sets

Barn-Burning Sprint Workouts

Strict Ring Dips
:10 on/:20 off
Accumulate 80 reps

C2 Bike
3 sets
:30 @ 335 watts
:30 easy

Assault Bike
2 rounds
Min 1: 15 cal Assault Bike
Min 2: 10 burpee bar touches
Min 3: 22 cal Assault Bike
Min 4: Rest

4

Coordination

I loved skiing growing up, but once I discovered the rush of the terrain park at Sugarbush Resort in Vermont, I switched from black diamond trails to doing crazy tricks whenever my family went to the slopes. That's where I was from the time we got to the mountain to the time we left, and I wouldn't even leave to eat lunch with my parents in the lodge.

But on one trip, the only way I could get in was if I entered the competition they were hosting that day, so I borrowed the $15 entry fee from my parents and signed up. Whether there were judges watching or not, I planned on doing what I always did: bombing it down the run as fast as possible and launching off the 70-foot kicker at the bottom. By this point, I was so comfortable throwing a backflip that I could do it off the bumps on the side of the trail, so that was the first trick I led off with.

I assumed that'd be enough to take first place. But right after me, another kid threw a backflip with a half twist. When I saw that from the chairlift, I knew I had to give myself a case of the "f——— its"—a seemingly crazy decision to try something new and probably a little reckless. And the trick I had in my mind was definitely a little reckless.

Even on the trampoline in our backyard, I'd never tried anything more advanced than a backflip, and I lost a bit of nerve when I entered the top of the terrain park. Still, I gassed myself up and skied down the mountain. *You can do it,* I thought. *You can do it.* Still, I had my doubts as I picked up speed, and even by the time I got to the start of the jump, I wasn't sure what I was about to do.

I took off the lip of the jump, tucked into a ball for my first backflip, and started to straighten my body. But as my head rotated around and I saw the ground, I fully committed to what I was doing. Without another thought, I pulled my knees into my chest, did another rotation, and just barely landed the second backflip upright. *Holy crap*, I thought. *I hope someone had that on camera.*

My parents weren't surprised, not that I went for the double or that I landed it. I'm lucky to have a lot of natural athleticism, and they'd seen the other ridiculous stunts I'd attempted. Still, they weren't happy about it and stared at me when I skied up to them afterward. "What were you thinking?"

If you want to be the best version of yourself, I don't recommend that you strap on your skis and go chuck a double. But I am a big proponent of the "f——— it" mentality. Especially when it comes to high-skill CrossFit movements, sometimes you need to act braver than you're feeling to get what you want—but only after you've put in the work and built a foundation.

WORKOUT: *Toddler Training*

10 Turkish Get-Ups

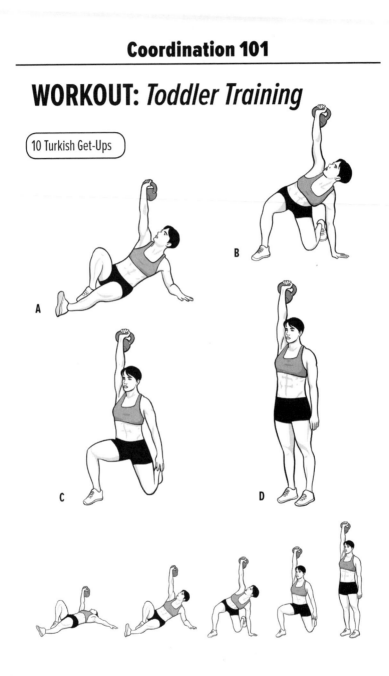

My parents were surprised when I stood up at six months old! At that age, babies are working on the stability to just sit on their own in a tripod position, but there I was, crawling and getting to my feet.

Three months later, I started walking, but I didn't have the coordination or strength to lower myself to the ground. Instead, I would timber straight back, whack my head on the carpet, then do it all over again. Eventually, my parents took a roll of foam and wrapped it around my head like a foam helmet. It was held together with a long sticker from my dad's real estate business so it looked like I had a name on my head. They would put this on my head when I got up each day and off I'd go.

As basic as it seems, being able to get off the ground and stand up is a great way to start improving your coordination, and the Turkish get-up will teach you two core principles. The first is how you can use tension to stabilize your body. That same technique is also how you'll eventually learn how to cycle your pull-ups in one fluid "butterfly" motion.

The second principle is how to keep your body aligned. Especially as you go up in weight with the Turkish get-up, you have to make sure the kettlebell in your hand is stacked on top of your shoulder, which is a position that will keep your joints safe in other movements, like handstand push-ups. So be diligent with your get-ups (foam helmet not necessary).

EXERCISE: *CrossFit Field Trip*

> Spend 15 minutes playing another sport

As I got older, I learned a lot of sports quickly. I swam across our 36-foot outdoor pool in one breath when I was four. I could walk for a dozen steps on my hands when I was seven. I was playing soccer, wrestling, Rollerblading, ice skating, and skiing double black diamonds by the time I was nine. CrossFit hadn't been invented yet, but even if it had, I'm not sure I would have benefited from starting that young.

With gyms offering classes especially for kids, and a teen division at the Games for athletes as young as fifteen, you're able to train CrossFit earlier and earlier. I think that's great, but it's also important to figure out what you like and what you don't. Both my parents were Olympic figure skaters for Canada. Naturally, I tried skating as a kid (I actually performed in my first ice show with them when I was four), but it wasn't for me, and my parents didn't push it.

When it came to quitting or changing sports, my parents only had one rule: Once we'd committed to something, we'd finish out that season. So I tried pretty much everything I could. What stuck was Olympic lifting (obviously), but I also played football, and I regret taking my junior year off from football so that I could train more weightlifting. Even if I wasn't destined for the NFL, I still loved playing, and it probably would've helped me at the Games. In fact, one of the main tenets of CrossFit is that you "regularly learn and play new sports," so try something new. Pick up surfing or golf or anything else that challenges you to move in unfamiliar ways and helps you avoid plateauing.

CrossFit Coordination 101

WORKOUT: *Flight Simulator*

Double-Unders
5, 10, 15, 20, 25, 30, 35, 40, 45, 50, 45, 40, 35, 30, 25, 20, 15, 10, 5

When I started CrossFit, I was lucky that I could already do most of the movements. Obviously I was familiar with the Olympic lifts, and I had the strength and body awareness to learn new skills, like a ring muscle-up, more or less on the first try. But there was something I couldn't do.

Like many of you, I'd jumped rope before but couldn't get the timing right for double-unders, so I asked our gym owner, Jade, for a workout to help me improve. He gave me the Flight Simulator. It's a workout with a huge volume of double-unders—500 total—but also has a catch: I had to do each set without making a mistake before moving on. As I walked to the back room of the gym, Jade told me not to try it for more than 10 minutes, which would be about 1,000 double-unders.

Around the 15-minute mark, Jade came back and stopped me. I hadn't finished, but I had done close to 1,500 jumps. I could barely walk the next day. But as soon as my calves recovered, I did the Flight Simulator every other day until I got it, about two weeks later. If you want to develop your coordination, the Flight Simulator is a great place to start because it trains your hand-eye coordination and your timing. Beware: Your calves will not be happy.

WORKOUT: *Pull-Up Progression 1*

12 Scap Push-Ups

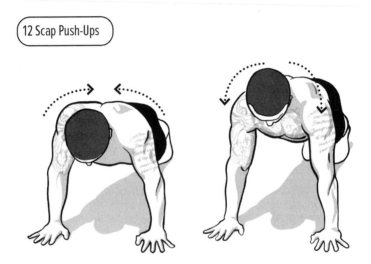

First, get into a plank position, with your hands directly underneath your shoulders, your toes touching the ground, and your body in one straight line (no sagging hips or butt in the air).

Careful: Even though this movement is called a push-up, the range of motion is much shorter. In fact, you should sink only a few inches, and your chest shouldn't be engaged at all.

Just like I did with deadlifting and rowing, I eventually sought out help with my gymnastics. This time, I went to Dave Durante, a multiple US national gymnastics champion, Stanford All-American gymnast, and co-owner of Power Monkey Fitness.

He told me that, no matter which upper-body movements you're doing, you're probably using your scapula (aka your shoulder blades). So you want to make sure that they're strong and mobile, and one of the best ways to do that is the scap push-up.

Look at the ground so your head is in a neutral position (i.e., aligned with the rest of your spine) and tighten your core so the only movement in your body comes from your shoulder blades. Keeping your arms straight and extended, and without bending your elbows, pinch an imaginary pencil between your shoulder blades. At first, it might be hard just to feel this part of your body, but that's okay. You'll get better with practice.

Now use your back muscles to push the ground away from you, creating space between your shoulder blades (that imaginary pencil should fall to the ground here). Hold that bottom position for a few seconds, trying to put as much distance as possible between your scapula. Then, using your back muscles again, pull the ground toward you and re-pinch the pencil between your shoulder blades. To make the movement easier, you can do the push-up standing against the wall or with your knees on the ground.

Scap push-ups are a great exercise that I incorporate into almost all my warm-ups, and once you've mastered them, you can move on to the next phase of the progression: strict pull-ups.

WORKOUT: *Pull-Up Progression 2*

10 Ring Rows
10 Banded Pull-Ups
10 Pull-Up Eccentrics

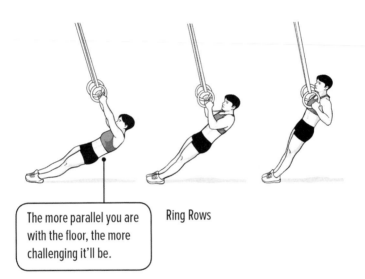

The more parallel you are with the floor, the more challenging it'll be.

Ring Rows

CrossFit has caught a lot of flak over the years for allowing kipping (when you use a swing to make the movement easier), and the most controversial movement is the kipping pull-up. A lot of the criticism about its being dangerous is wrong (I've done thousands of kipping pull-ups without injuring my shoulders), but I do think too many of you start to kip way too early. You need a certain base level of strength in your arms and shoulders, and if you aren't able to do at least one strict pull-up, you definitely aren't ready to swing.

There are a lot of progressions to help you get that first pull-up.

Pull-Up Progression 2 (Cont.)

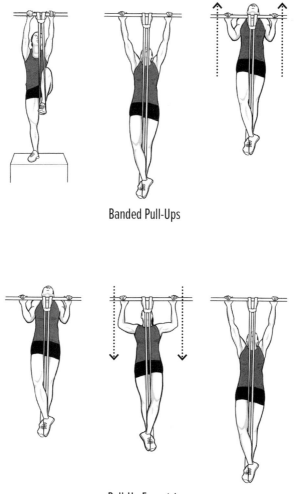

Banded Pull-Ups

Pull-Up Eccentrics

One of them is ring rows. Find a set of rings, check that they're about as wide as your shoulders, and position your body underneath them. Then pull up, making sure that you squeeze your shoulder blades together (just like at the top of that scap push-up), that you stay in a hollow position and don't arch your back, and that you finish the movement with the bottom of the rings touching your chest.

Another progression is banded pull-ups. You're going to hook an elastic band around the pull-up bar so that there's a loop at the bottom for your knee or your foot.

This variation is helpful because it teaches your body what the movement is supposed to feel like, but it's not my favorite way to learn. It's hard to find a band that gives you the right amount of support, so I prefer practicing eccentrics, when you jump up above the bar and then lower yourself down as slowly as possible. This is actually where you build the most strength, so try to resist gravity as much as you can here.

Learning to do a pull-up strict may take longer than you'd like, especially when you have to scale the workout to ring rows whereas everyone else at your gym does it as prescribed, but eventually you'll have the foundation you need to move on to the next skill: kipping.

Kipping is a movement that's easy to do wrong, especially when you're tired. Remember: The more tension you create in your body, the more power you produce, so swinging isn't an excuse to slack off and relax.

But before you can add the pull-up to your kip, you have to learn the proper body positions. So lie on the ground faceup. Then press your lower back into the ground and raise up your shoulders and toes. No matter what, you should feel this almost exclusively

WORKOUT: *Pull-Up Progression 3*

3 Sets
00:30 Hollow Hold
10 Beat Swings

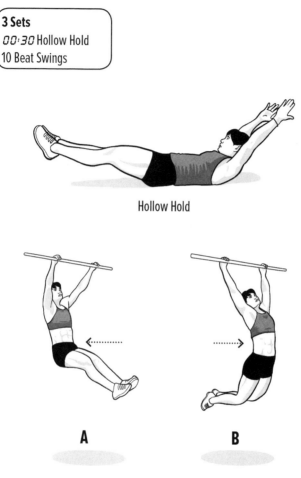

Hollow Hold

A

B

Beat Swings

in your abs and definitely not in your lower back. This is a "hollow" position, what you need to hit at the back of your kip swing.

Next, stay on the ground and lie facedown with your arms

straight above your head. Then raise your torso, shoulders, and arms, along with your quads and toes. All that should be left on the ground is your core and pelvis, and you should aim to make your body as long as possible, like it's being pulled from the top and bottom. That's the position you want to hit at the front of your kip swing.

Next, practice hanging. Hop onto the bar and initiate an "active" hang by pulling your scaps down and squeezing your quads and glutes. Your body should be in one straight line and your neck should be a little longer than usual. If this is a difficult position to hold, or if your grip is giving out almost immediately, you need to practice hanging before moving on to swinging.

Then you're ready to swing. Starting in a dead hang, pull your chest forward and your feet backward so you end up looking like a backward "C," aka that second hollow position from the floor. As you swing backward, return to the hollow position but with your hands and feet a little farther in front of you, so you end up in that first hollow position from the floor. At both ends of the swing, your entire body should be in one curve, which shows that your upper and lower body are working in unison to create a single action. If there are any sharp angles, it can lead to slack and put too much stress on your joints.

As you get more comfortable with the arch and hollow, you can swing farther in each direction in preparation for the kipping pull-up. However, most people swing more than they are capable of handling, so only swing within a range where the elbows are always locked out.

WORKOUT: *Pull-Up Progression 4*

3 Sets
5 Kipping Pull-Ups
5 Toes-to-Bars

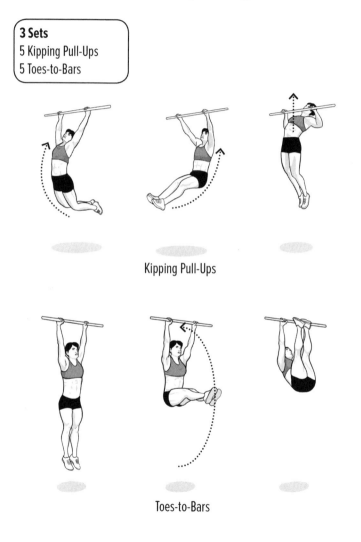

Kipping Pull-Ups

Toes-to-Bars

Once you've got the beat swing, practice pushing down on the bar during your backswing. It sounds counterintuitive, but that's how you transfer the power from the kip into the pull-up. If you relax your arms and go limp on the backswing, you'll lose all your momentum. But if you stay engaged and keep that tension in your body until you're at the top of the swing, you'll be able to pull up the rest of the way and get your chin over the bar.

Getting your first kipping pull-up is an exciting moment, but the real accomplishment is stringing them together, which takes a bit more work. You have to do everything in reverse; most important, pushing down on the bar as you swing down. Otherwise, you lose all the tension and power you just built and have to start the next beat swing from scratch. So as you practice, try to string together as many kipping pull-ups as possible while still maintaining perfect form. But remember: Don't swing more than you can handle. If your elbows start to bend, your swing is out of control.

Thankfully, you'll have more opportunities to practice because this is the same movement you use when you do toes-to-bars. Again, I think you should be able to do one strict toes-to-bar before you start to kip, but if you jump straight to kipping, use that same beat swing: Hit the backward "C" position in the front by initiating the movement with your shoulders, leading with your chest, and keeping tension in your scaps, glutes, and quads. Then get into the frontward "C" position by pulling down on the bar, squeezing your abs, and keeping your feet together. When you're at the top of your backswing, kick your feet up instead of pulling your chin over the bar to finish the toe-to-bar.

The more efficiently you can kip, the easier it will be to transition to the "butterfly" method, the most efficient way to do pull-ups.

WORKOUT: *Pull-Up Progression 5*

3 Sets
10 Butterfly Pull-Ups

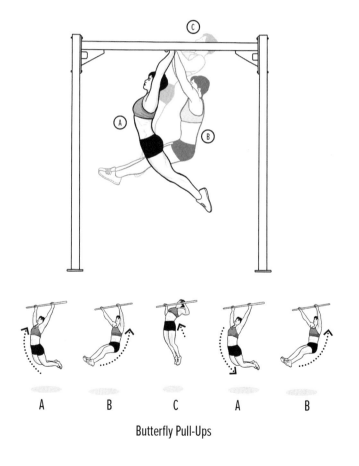

Butterfly Pull-Ups

Butterfly may look way different from the kip, but it's actually more or less the same. You're still going to alternate between the arched "C" and hollow positions, but instead of pulling up so you hit the top of your swing when your chin is directly above the bar, you pull a bit earlier, so you're at your highest point a few inches behind the bar. That way, you can continue swinging forward and underneath the bar in an oval movement. Then when you're at the end of your "C" position, kick your legs toward the bar and push down to transition back to the arched position.

It sounds complicated, but if you did your homework with the kipping pull-ups, you have all the ingredients you need. Two important things to remember. First: Just like with double-unders, timing is everything, and it takes practice to learn exactly when to push and pull on the bar and when to kick your legs forward. You might want to stand on a box and practice the movement before you attempt it swinging.

Second: Because butterflies are one continuous swing, there's a lot more stress on your shoulders, meaning it's even more important that you strengthen your scaps and all the stabilizing muscles in your shoulders.

So tread slowly through this progression. I know it's easy to get impatient when you see the other athletes at your gym blowing through huge sets of butterfly pull-ups, and you're still doing ring rows. But trust me, it isn't worth going a few seconds faster and destroying your rotator cuff in the process. And the good news is that once you've perfected the butterfly method for pull-ups, you've basically got it down for chest-to-bars, too. You'll just need a little more strength.

WORKOUT: *Handstand Progression 1*

3 Sets
00:30 Wall-Facing Handstand Holds

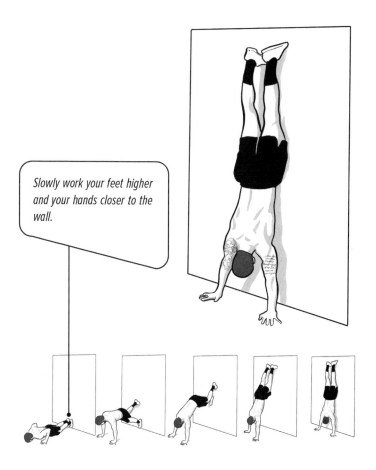

Slowly work your feet higher and your hands closer to the wall.

It's relatively easy to do an ugly handstand. Just put your hands on the ground, kick your feet up, and flail around until you come crashing down. If you're just messing around at the beach, that's all well and good, but if you want to train something like deficit handstand push-ups and not obliterate your shoulders in the process, you've got to have good technique. To do a wall walk, start in a push-up position with your feet against the wall and then walk your hands toward your toes and climb your feet up the wall. The goal is to end up completely vertical against the wall, but remember that a handstand isn't all or nothing, and if you aren't comfortable getting from the floor to the wall and back down, it can get ugly. So walk your feet up only as far as you can control (including the descent, too). With each step, you should be able to pause and hold that position.

As always, you want your core engaged and to activate your scaps and push through the ground. You don't want the force of gravity to shove your shoulders into your ears.

Slowly work your feet higher and your hands closer to the wall, and at the very top, touch your nose to the wall, just like you practiced with the holds from the last section. This last part is particularly important because you can have perfect body awareness when you're right side up, but a lot of people lose it the second they go upside down.

To end up against the wall, you have to be in one straight line, with your ankles over your knees over your hips over your shoulders over your hands.

If your spine is curved and overextended, like it probably will be at the beginning, you won't be able to touch your nose to the

WORKOUT: *Handstand Progression 2*

3 Rounds
3 Wall Walks

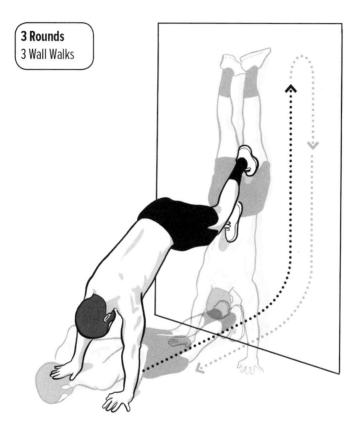

cinder blocks, which is the goal. If you find that you are an upside-down banana, squeeze your core and "tuck" your hips underneath you, like you did for the hollow holds on the ground.

It shouldn't surprise you that I recommend learning a strict handstand push-up before doing it kipping, and you should use more or less the same progressions as from the pull-ups. Eccentrics

WORKOUT: *Handstand Progression 3*

> **3 Rounds**
> 3 Pike Push-Ups
> 3 Handstand Push-Up Eccentrics

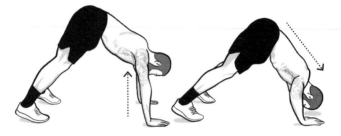

Pike Push-Ups

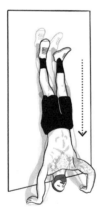

> *Eccentrics are a great way to build strength, as long as you're able to do them slow and controlled and with good body positioning.*

Handstand Push-Up Eccentrics

are a great way to build strength, as long as you're able to do them slow and controlled and with good body positioning. If you don't yet have that strength, or if you're nervous about crashing to the ground, stack ab mats underneath your head.

Another great coordination-building exercise you can do is pike push-ups, which are like a normal push-up, but with your hips high in the air. The same principle applies here as it did with ring rows—the more vertical your hips get, the harder it is. So start with your feet on the ground. Then as you build strength, put them on a higher and higher surface so that your torso is in one vertical line. If your hamstrings are especially tight, you can bend your knees to get into that stacked vertical position.

Regardless of which exercise you're doing, your head should always land a little in front of your hands, so the three points make a triangle, and if you had to, you'd be able to balance on your head. When you've eventually got the strength and stability to do a vertical pike push-up, you're ready to do a strict handstand push-up.

The movement should look like this: You're at the top of a handstand with your back facing the wall, pushing against the ground using your shoulders. Then you lower yourself so your head's on the ground. Your head and neck should be neutral (looking ahead and not up or down), and your hands should be a little farther away from the wall so that they form that triangle with your head.

Without using your legs or hips at all, push your head off the ground and return to your original starting position. Your heels

WORKOUT: *Handstand Progression 4*

AMRAP
Strict Handstand Push-Ups

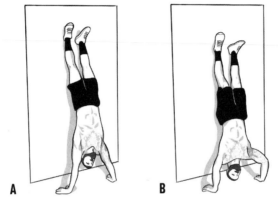

A   **B**

Strict Handstand Push-Ups

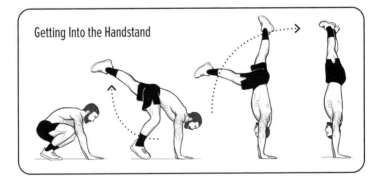

Getting Into the Handstand

should be just as high as they were when you started. If they aren't, you're likely overextending as you push up and need to work more on hollow holds and building shoulder strength. But if you're able to do a few reps cleanly, congratulations, you can kip.

Nothing changes until you get to the bottom of the handstand, when you're balancing on your hands and your head in that triangle position. That's when you lower your knees down toward your elbows. Then as you push with your hands, you kick your legs up like you're trying to break a ceiling right above you. That extra momentum from your hips should make the movement easier, but don't let it compromise your body positioning. Are your heels still above that line? Don't guess. For all these movements, set up your phone and film yourself to make sure.

From there, the next skill is walking on your hands, which is a bit scarier. It's already awkward to be upside down, let alone to fall forward and catch yourself. But you have to ignore the worst-case scenario and give it your all, which is something I learned from my parents.

While my parents were warming up for their first big pairs figure skating competition, my mom was in a lift above my dad's head when he caught a toe pick, tripped, and threw her onto the ice, cracking her pelvis. Still she refused to withdraw from the Canadian championships six weeks later. Not only did she do the same lift there, but they also won the silver medal.

Learning new skills, especially the gymnastics ones, can be intimidating, but you can practice working through your fear. That's why I recommend learning the handstand forward roll.

WORKOUT: *Building Confidence*

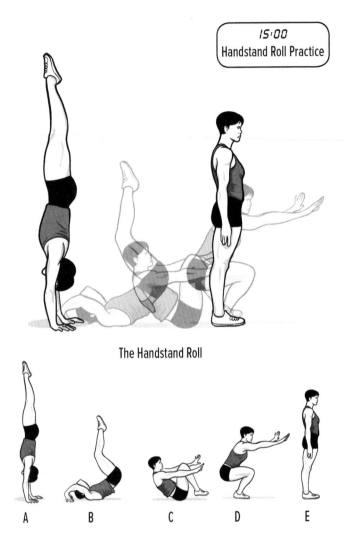

15:00
Handstand Roll Practice

The Handstand Roll

A   B   C   D   E

First, start by finding a soft surface and getting into a crouched position with your hands on the ground. Then tuck your chin, which will curve your spine, and slowly lower your head to the ground. At this point, your weight will be carrying you forward, and if you give a slight jump (and keep your chin tucked), you'll roll over onto your back. As you get more comfortable with this forward roll, you can initiate the jump earlier, making sure to keep your chin tucked.

Then, when you're in the handstand, have someone grab your ankles and hold you as you bend your arms, lower yourself toward the ground, and tuck your chin so you roll onto your back. Practicing that skill with confidence will help you do the same with more intimidating movements.

With a solid handstand in your wheelhouse, you've mastered most of the gymnastics moves in CrossFit. Now you can start to refine them.

WORKOUT: *Gripapalooza*

3 Sets
1:00 Dead Hang
50-foot Farmer's Carry
50-foot Plate Pinches

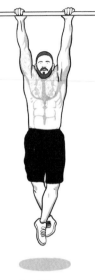

Dead Hang

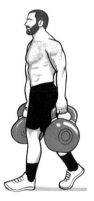

Farmer's Carry

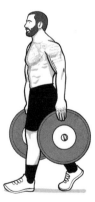

Plate Pinches

If you want to get a better snatch, you don't train the one-rep max every day, and it's the same with kipping movements. You might get a little more efficient if you practice them each workout, but there's a quick plateau.

For that reason, I typically choose not to do any kipping movements for most of the season. Especially at the beginning of my career, I was more focused on building that base level of strength, so I waited until two or three weeks before competition before I'd start familiarizing myself with the kipping motion again.

By going strict, I realized that my grip was the reason I couldn't do monster sets of pull-ups, so I practiced dead hangs, farmer carries, and plate pinches to improve. Then I noticed that my hand dexterity sucked after I'd hop off the bar. That sounds like a minor problem, but it's not if you have to transition to another movement, like a handstand walk. I've seen so many people land on their own fingers and trip because they couldn't open their hands enough. So I practiced obliterating my forearms until they were big and puffy, then I'd go straight into handstand walks.

You could see that work pay off in Friendly Fran, the first workout of the 2020 Games. It was three rounds of 21 thrusters and 21 chest-to-bars, and I finished in 3:08, 47 seconds faster than the second-place guy and at a pace of one rep every second and a half.

There was a lot of work that went into making that event a success, but something you might not notice is that I opened my hands wide after finishing each set of chest-to-bars. That way, I could slide my hands onto the barbell in exactly the position I wanted instead of trying to open my hands at the last second and

WORKOUT: *Ring Muscle-Up Progression 1*

3 Sets
5 Strict Chest-to-Bar Ring Pull-Ups
5 Dips
5 Banded Muscle-Up Transitions

Use False Grip

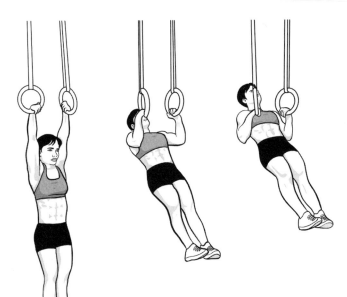

Strict Chest-to-Bar Ring Pull-Ups

Ring Muscle-Up Progression 1 (Cont.)

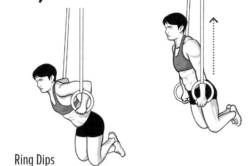

Ring Dips

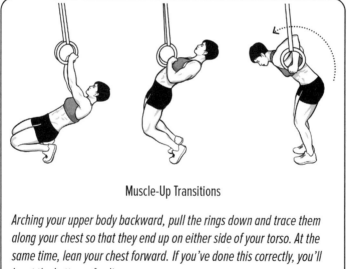

Muscle-Up Transitions

Arching your upper body backward, pull the rings down and trace them along your chest so that they end up on either side of your torso. At the same time, lean your chest forward. If you've done this correctly, you'll be at the bottom of a dip.

risking catching my pinkie on the bar. That wouldn't be a huge time drain, possibly half a second, but maybe it would've hurt, and probably I would've panicked a little. No matter what, it would've taken up mental space, like *Oh no, I made a mistake*. So why take the risk?

The last major gymnastics skill is the muscle-up. Because it's harder to do on the rings than the bar, that's what I'll focus on.

But before we get to the kipping muscle-up, yeah, that's right, we're going to learn how to do it strict. But don't worry. You already know all the fundamentals, except for two things. The first is the dip, which is the last part of the movement. If a dip isn't currently in your wheelhouse, practice the eccentric to build that strength and the depth awareness (your shoulders should be touching the top of the rings).

The second is the grip. To make it easier to transition between the two parts of the movement—the initial pull-up on the rings and then the dip on top of them—you'll need the rings to slide in your hands. That requires a false grip, and the easiest way to get it is to do this: Grab the side of the rings that's farthest from you and grip it like you're holding on to a pole. Then rotate the ring toward the ground. Your hand should now be positioned so that the bottom of your wrist is resting on the rings. It's going to be uncomfortable at first, but you can get used to it by hanging in the false grip.

Using that false grip, do a chest-to-bar and pull the rings as far down on your torso as possible. That'll make it easier to do the next part, the transition.

This is an especially tricky transition at first, so now is when I would recommend using a band. Tie it between a squatting rig so it creates a seat underneath the rings. That way you can practice the transition without getting exhausted after the first rep. The focus here is on technique, so take plenty of rest and don't rush the movement. The slower you're able to do this, the easier it will be to do the eccentric.

To prepare for the eccentric, set the rings at a height where you can touch the ground when you're at the bottom of a dip.

Like with the pull-up and handstand push-up eccentric, you're going to do the movement in reverse. Start on top of the rings, with your arms straight like you've just finished a dip. Then lower yourself down until you can use your legs to take some of the weight off your arms. After that, work your way through the transition as carefully as possible, bringing the rings from your sides into the middle of your chest. When you finish this step, your hands should be in that false grip position. Then you can let go of the rings and start another rep.

Once you've mastered these two exercises, all that's left is to put them together. You're probably going to get caught at the transition, and that's okay. If there's someone around who can spot you, have them support your hips when you can't pull the rings any farther, just like how you used the elastic band. And when you get to the top, resist the urge to drop off the rings and start celebrating. The slower you can control your descent, the more strength you'll build. Then you're ready to start kipping. But first, a warning.

WORKOUT: *Ring Muscle-Up Progression 2*

> **3 Sets**
> 5 Muscle-Up Eccentrics
> As many Ring Muscle-Ups as possible

Use False Grip

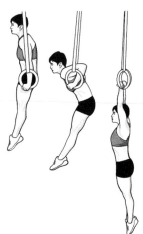

Ring Muscle-Up Eccentrics

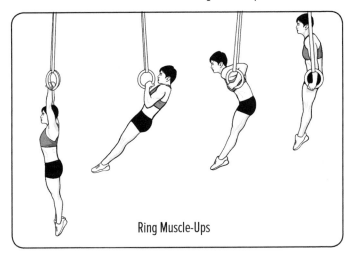

Ring Muscle-Ups

CrossFit Games Coordination

A kipping ring muscle-up is a serious movement, and your body should be prepared for it. Obviously everyone's different, but a general gauge is that you should be able to dead hang for at least a minute, do three strict pull-ups, and five strict dips.

However, when it comes to technique, you've already got everything you need if you've been doing your homework from the earlier chapters. Even though the swing is on the rings, not on a bar, it's a more exaggerated version of the hollow and arch positions that you know. Practice that swing so that you can do it perfectly, with no slack in your body at any point. Then since you've also mastered the dip, what's left is the scariest part: the transition.

Instead of being slow and controlled, you need to be dynamic and confident here. It's best to practice it first, so pull out your elastic band again and set it up on the squat rig at about hip height. You should be able to lie faceup with your butt on the band and your hands on the rings at about an 80-degree angle. This is exactly how you want to feel at the top of your swing— parallel with the ground (no sagging hips) and pulling down on the rings. From there, get a little bounce from the band and pull your torso forward like you're trying to headbutt a soccer ball. Your shoulders should travel over the rings, not through them, and you should end with your eyes forward, your elbows back, and the rings pressed into your torso. And during the entire movement, work to keep the rings as close to you as possible.

You want to practice that banded transition until it's second nature, and only then should you try it without the band. From

WORKOUT: *Ring Muscle-Up Progression 3*

> **As many reps as FORM allows**
> Kipping Ring Muscle-Ups

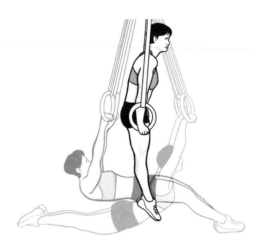

Kipping Ring Muscle-Ups

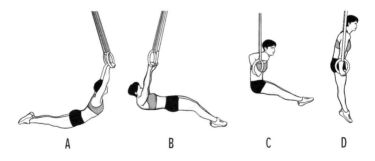

A   B   C   D

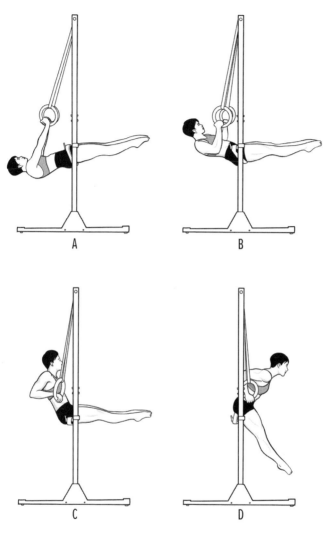

A   B

C   D

Banded Muscle-Up Transitions

WORKOUT: *Ring Around the World*

3 Sets
3 Kipping Ring Muscle-Ups, each set at different strap lengths

Short Length

Medium Length

Long Length

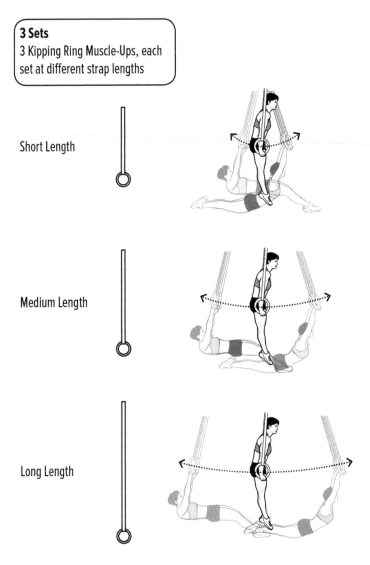

there, you can learn to cycle your reps and modify your technique based on the strap length, but it helps to understand a little bit of physics first.

You think a muscle-up is a muscle-up, but there's a huge difference in the movement depending on how long the rings' straps are, their material, what they're anchored to, and even the width of the rings and whether they're made of metal or wood.

What you want to see is three-quarter-inch wood rings connected to short straps that are made out of cloth and attached to a shrimp trawler, the metal bar that hangs out over a normal squatting rig. This is the easiest they'll ever get and a good way to learn the movement.

What you don't want, above all else, is long, 25-foot straps, like the ones hanging from the Zeus rig at the 2018 Games. I don't care if you'd done 30 ring muscle-ups every day for a year, that was an entirely different workout. Still, a lot of guys swung with the cadence they always use in the gym, and some of their timing was totally off because the straps were so long. They paid the price. If you start doing your kip while the rings are swung forward, you're going to get off cadence and start to swing like a pendulum. Now you have to kip even more because the rings are higher, but if you wait to kip until the rings are swinging back, they're going to be underneath you at the top of your swing.

If your gym has multiple sets of rings, use them all to learn how to better control your swing and timing. And if your gym doesn't, lengthen and shorten the straps as much as you can, or make it a point to try out the rings when you visit a new gym.

WORKOUT: *The Pegboard*

3 Pegboard Ascents

The farther you lean away from the pegs, the more your weight is distributed to your feet and not your hands. Otherwise, you're basically doing a dead-hang strict pull-up every time you want to move up.

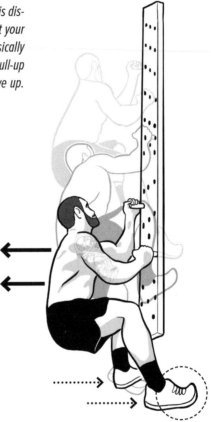

Like I said before, the essence of the Games is that they're "unknown and unknowable." The events themselves are a secret, but that doesn't mean there aren't patterns. We know there's going

Hard Work Pays Off

to be a swim and a run. And we know there'll be heavy lifting, like the CrossFit Total, a one-rep max on the snatch, or a clean speed ladder.

But even if there's an entirely new event, you can be prepared by understanding a little bit about force and gravity.

That's what helped me when the pegboard was introduced at the 2015 Games. I was in the last heat, so I watched the other guys from a TV in the athlete area, and my hands were sweating. No one could figure it out. They'd get a few feet off the ground and then slide back down or hang from the pegs long enough to get totally gassed and drop off. I was nervous I'd do the same, but I was also convinced that they were approaching it all wrong.

For one, most were wearing shoes with an aggressive sole, which was insane. Have you ever seen someone try to walk on concrete with cleats? It's almost impossible because the rubber spikes only work if they're digging into a soft surface, like dirt. If you really want to get traction on something completely flat, like the plexiglass wall, you need another flat surface, ideally one with as much surface area as possible, so I was one of the only guys on the field wearing his lifting shoes.

Next, I knew it would be easiest if I pushed myself away from the wall. Especially as you get higher off the ground, it's a natural reaction to lean in close to the wall, and that's the advice that the commentators were giving. But I knew that was wrong from studying engineering.

That doesn't mean my strategy was perfect that year. I was the fourth one off the pegboard, but I was happy with how I was able to apply what I knew about physics to a new situation.

The Coordination Mentality

JOURNAL ENTRY—What are your pre-workout routines? Are there any consistent sights, sounds, or smells that you rely on? How do you visualize yourself at your most important moment? What are you wearing, hearing, and doing?

Same as someone putting on their suit to go to work, I have a routine that lets my body and mind know that I'm going to compete. I visualize myself walking out onto the floor, hearing the noise of the crowd, and feeling the energy in the stadium. And the final event at the 2019 Games was no different.

This one was an absolute slog: 30 clean and jerks (Grace), followed by 30 ring muscle-ups, followed by 30 snatches (Isabel). It was too long to sprint and too short to cruise. And unlike the two previous years, my lead over the other guys wasn't insurmountable. In fact, if Noah Ohlsen and one other guy beat me, he would win. But I had something he didn't: the DJ for the CrossFit Games.

Every year before the final event, Sammy texted the DJ and asked him to play my theme song for that year of training. I didn't know that Sammy had asked him to do it the first time, and I was the last one in the tunnel before going down the flight of stairs and walking into the arena. There were people to the right and left of me, and I was already emotional because I knew that I'd won. But then I heard "Old Thing Back," with Biggie Smalls, Matoma, and Ja Rule. This was what I listened to every day on the drive to the gym, and just knowing that Sammy thought to request it made me start crying.

This year, in the tunnel before the last event of the 2019 Games, I heard Queen's "We Will Rock You." This was a deep cut, the song I'd start when I was exactly three and a half minutes away from Champlain Valley CrossFit and was ready to blow out my speakers. That was when I'd picture myself at the Games, with the lights on and the crowd going wild. And here was that moment, with the arena shaking as 30,000 fans *boom-boom-clapped* along with the song. *They're doing that for you,* I told myself. *They're here to watch you win. They didn't show up to see you take second place.* I was ready to run through a wall.

I'm sorry, guys, I thought when I jogged onto the floor and over to my lane. *I'm winning the workout. Like, you can do whatever you want, but I'm winning.* And then I looked up to see Ohlsen. He had his eyes closed and was doing the boom-boom-clap above his head. *Sorry, bro,* I thought. *This song is for me.*

I was so jacked up for that workout that if I'd had to PR my 2-kilometer row at the start, I felt like I still would've won it.

So what can you draw on that takes you to that mental place? Is it a song? An image? A specific memory? What can you incorporate into your daily training that guides you toward one specific moment, so that when you get there, you're absolutely amped?

Eating for Coordination

I wish Sammy had a recipe to make you better at handstand push-ups and kipping ring muscle-ups, but sadly, there's no food I know of that improves your coordination. However, fitting enough nutritious meals into your training schedule does require a lot of logistical coordination.

Even though Sammy loves to cook, she's got her own life going on. She's a boss influencer, a cookbook author, and a pretty decent Olympic lifter herself, so she doesn't want to spend her entire day in the kitchen. Especially when she had to feed me, Tia, and Shane, she wants to be as efficient as possible—and I imagine you do, too.

Overnight Oats

1 cup old-fashioned oats

$1^{1}/_{2}$ cups coconut milk

2 ripe bananas, mashed

$^{1}/_{4}$ cup plain Greek yogurt

2 tablespoons maple syrup

1 tablespoon chia seeds

2 teaspoons vanilla

$^{1}/_{4}$ teaspoon flaky salt

Fruit, nuts, maple syrup, granola, etc., for serving (optional)

1. In a large bowl, stir together the oats, milk, bananas, yogurt, maple syrup, chia seeds, vanilla, and salt. Divide among 4 mason jars. Cover and refrigerate overnight.
2. To serve, in the morning, stir and add the toppings of your choice: sliced bananas, strawberries, fresh jam, nuts/nut butters, maple syrup, granola, etc. The possibilities are endless!

I'm sure you've heard it a million times, but preparation is key. Even though we eat a ton of food when I'm in season—we go through a five-pound bag of rice every other week—Sammy goes to the store only two or three times a week. She knows exactly what we need, and she'd go even less if she weren't buying so many fresh foods, which usually spoil within a few days. So keep a list of what you're eating (and what's ending up in the trash), and know the meals you're going to make for the next few days. Especially if you aren't a morning person, like me, make sure your breakfast is ready to go the night before. Otherwise, it's easy to skip it altogether and watch your workouts suffer.

Cinny-Sweet Peanut Butter Toast

2 slices sourdough bread, toasted

2 to 4 tablespoons peanut butter (mine had sea salt and chia seeds mixed in)

1 to 2 teaspoons honey

1 teaspoon cinnamon

Double shot of espresso for serving (optional)

1. Smear the toasted bread with the peanut butter.
2. Drizzle the peanut butter toast with the honey and sprinkle with the cinnamon.
3. Enjoy with a double shot of espresso, if desired, for a perfect morning pairing.

Also work smart and hard. One of Sammy's secret weapons is a slow cooker, which gives you the freedom to throw in all the ingredients, spend a few hours at the gym, and come back to a full meal. Whether it's making mass quantities of foods that freeze easily, or cooking up sides that can be added to pretty much anything, optimize your time in the kitchen. While there are some things you can do while multitasking, like chopping onions and stirring stews, it's typically best to set aside an hour or two each week and focus exclusively on prep.

Simple Roasted Beets

6 to 8 beets

2 tablespoons olive oil

Pinch of flaky kosher salt

1. Preheat the oven to 425°F.
2. Scrub the beets under cold running water and pat dry with a towel. Drizzle with the olive oil and season with salt.
3. Wrap the beets in aluminum foil and place on a baking sheet in the oven to roast for 40 to 60 minutes (depending on their size) until fork tender.
4. Allow the roasted beets to cool slightly before running under cold water to remove the skin.
5. Season with salt, slice, and serve.

I'm notoriously bad about eating leftovers, so Sammy typically eats whatever we haven't finished from the night before, or she converts it into another full meal. For example, if she's cooking steak, she always makes me two. If I only eat one and a half, she cooks the rest into a steak hash the next day. If you're creative with your leftovers, you can cook more than you need and not worry about wasting.

Crispy Carnitas

4 pounds pork butt (or shoulder)

3 to 4 teaspoons salt

1 teaspoon pepper

1 tablespoon dried oregano (or Mexican oregano)

1 tablespoon ground cumin

1 large sweet onion, diced

8 cloves garlic, smashed

2 limes, juiced

3 large oranges, 2 juiced/1 sliced

2 bay leaves

1 or 2 tablespoons olive oil

1. Rinse and pat dry the pork with a paper towel.
2. To a slow cooker, add the pork, salt, pepper, oregano, cumin, onion, garlic, lime juice, orange juice, and bay leaves.
3. Cover and cook on LOW for 8 to 10 hours, or HIGH for 5 to 6 hours (until the meat falls apart).
4. Remove the pork from the slow cooker (do not discard the liquid; reserve for use later) and shred with two forks on a plate.
5. Heat 1 tablespoon of the oil in a cast-iron skillet over high heat. When the pan is hot, add half of the shredded pork, searing until just beginning to crisp. Ladle over $1/2$ cup of the reserved liquid and continue cooking until the juices begin to reduce down and the meat is nice and crispy. Remove the cooked pork to a plate and repeat the process to cook the remaining batch, using more oil and reserved liquid if needed.

When finished, return the first batch of cooked pork to the skillet and mix to combine. Remove the skillet from the heat. Enjoy!

Even if you love to cook, sometimes it's worth paying a little extra to avoid some of the grunt work. For example, you can get vegetables that were picked at their peak of ripeness, chopped, and frozen. Reheating them requires a little practice—try to let them thaw for a bit, then put them in the microwave and cook them on low to medium heat—but it's easier than starting from scratch. If you do go for the fresh vegetables, avoid preparing them en masse unless they take a long time to cook, like sweet potatoes. If it's something simple, like the three minutes it takes to steam broccoli, Sammy will do it fresh for each meal.

Garlic Brown Butter Lobster Ramen

3 brown rice ramen noodle packs (seasoning discarded)

6 tablespoons salted butter

4 cloves garlic, grated

$1/_2$ lemon, sliced

8 ounces ButcherBox lobster claw meat

2 tablespoons fresh chives, chopped

1. Fill a large pot with water and cook the ramen according to the package instructions. Drain and set aside.
2. Heat a large cast-iron pan over medium heat. Add the butter to brown for 2 to 3 minutes until foamy and fragrant. To the brown butter, add the garlic and lemon slices. Cook, stirring, for an additional 2 minutes. Add the lobster. Cook for 3 to 5 minutes, stirring continuously.
3. Add the ramen to the pan, remove from the heat, and toss to combine. Sprinkle with the chopped chives and serve immediately.

When it comes to eating outside your house, Tupperware is your biggest ally. Have your meals packed and ready, so all you have to do in the morning is stuff them into your bag and walk out the door. As for what to cook, a lot of gyms and offices have a refrigerator and microwave, and some combination of rice, veggies, and meat is an easy meal to reheat. If you don't have access to either, you might want to think about sandwiches. There are some really healthy breads and cold cuts out there, and it's worth putting in the effort to find what works best for you.

Korean Beef Bowls

2 tablespoons olive oil, divided

1 pound ground beef

3 garlic cloves, minced

2 tablespoons maple syrup

$1/4$ cup tamari (or soy sauce)

2 teaspoons sesame oil

$1/4$ teaspoon ground ginger

$1/4$ teaspoon crushed red pepper flakes

$1/4$ teaspoon pepper

2 large eggs

2 cups cooked white rice

Sliced green onions and sesame seeds for serving

1. In a large skillet, heat 1 tablespoon of the olive oil over medium heat. When the oil shimmers, add the ground beef and cook until no pink remains. Add the garlic and cook an additional 2 minutes, stirring often to fully incorporate.

2. In a small bowl, mix the maple syrup, tamari, sesame oil, ginger, red pepper flakes, and pepper. Pour the sauce over the ground beef in the skillet and simmer 1 to 2 minutes until the beef is fully coated. Remove the pan from the heat and set aside until ready to assemble.

3. In a separate small skillet, heat the remaining 1 tablespoon oil over medium heat. Crack the eggs into the pan and cook until your desired doneness (I suggest sunny-side up and oozy yolk!).

4. To assemble your bowl, add the cooked white rice as your base and top with the sauced beef and fried egg. Sprinkle with sliced green onions and sesame seeds to serve.

Additional Coordination Training

WORKOUT:

3 Sets
5/5 World's greatest stretch
15 Hip Extensions
:20 L sit Hold

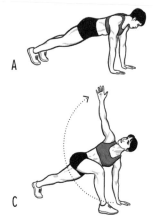

A

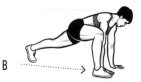

B

C

D

World's Greatest Stretch

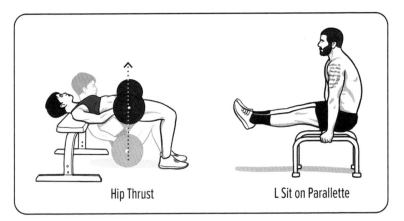

Hip Thrust   L Sit on Parallette

WORKOUT

3 Sets
25 Shoulder Taps

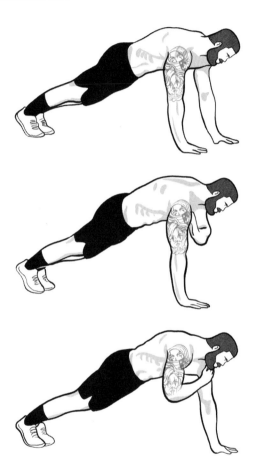

WORKOUT

4 Rounds
2:30 work, *1:00* rest
25 Hand Release Push-Ups
20 Jumping Air Squats
5 V-Ups
Max Burpees

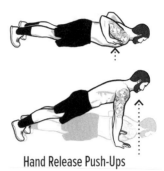

Hand Release Push-Ups

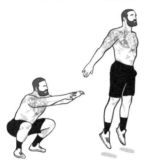

Jumping Air Squats

V-Ups

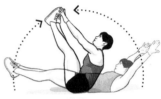

Burpees

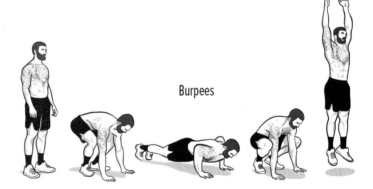

Handstand

3 Sets of 2 rounds
60 double-unders
15 strict handstand push-ups
10/10m dumbbell walking lunge
(heavy)
Rest: 2 mins between sets

Every 3 mins for 5 sets
(with vest)
8″ deficit handstand push-ups
Rest: 30 secs
2 strict muscle-ups +
5 muscle-ups

EMOM for 10 mins
1 m handstand walk over plates

27–21–15–9
Strict handstand push-ups
Box jump 24″

Conditioning

WORKOUT

Every *2:30* **for 4 sets**
2 L-Sit Rope Climbs
15 Chest-Supported Dumbbell Rows

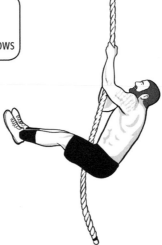

L-Sit Rope Climb

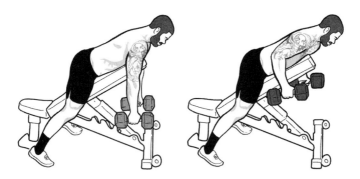

Chest-Supported Dumbbell Row

WORKOUT

Accumulate Max L-Sit Hold in 2:00

WORKOUT

Weighted Plank Hold
Accumulate 5:00 16 kg

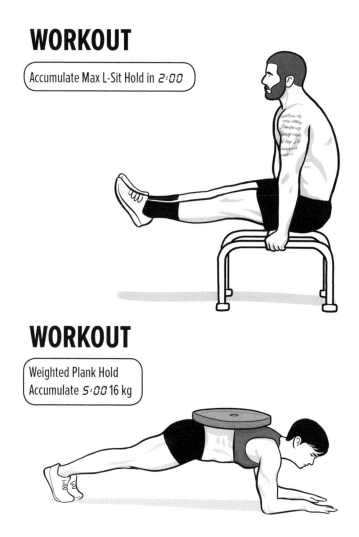

For time
1 mile run
100 ft handstand walk
10 burpee box get-overs 48″

1 mile run
100 ft handstand walk
10 burpee box get-overs
1 mile run (with vest or ruck)

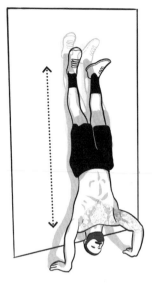

WORKOUT

Every _3:00_ **for 4 sets**
15 Strict Handstand Push-Ups
10 Hip Thrust
10L/10R Standing Oblique

Strict Handstand Push-Ups

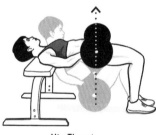

Hip Thrust

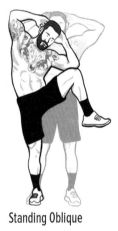

Standing Oblique

WORKOUT

Every _3:00_ **for 4 sets**
25 Ring Dips
15 Dumbbell Romanian Deadlifts
25 Push-Ups

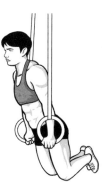
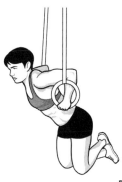

Ring Dips

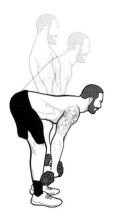

Dumbbell Romanian Deadlift

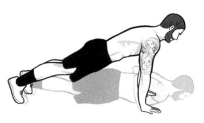

Push-Ups

WORKOUT

3 Sets
15 Hip Thrusts
10 Scap Pull-Ups
5 Inchworms

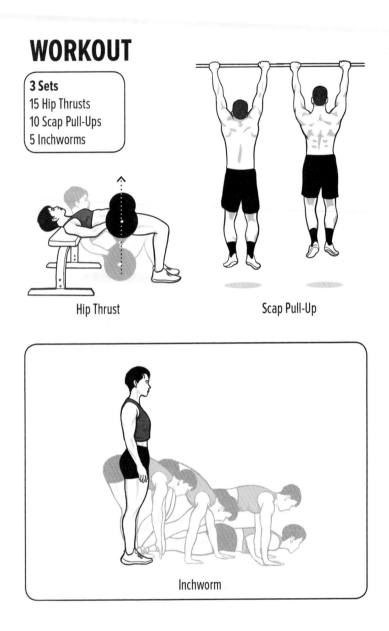

Hip Thrust

Scap Pull-Up

Inchworm

Weighted Ring Dips

5 × 5

Every 3 mins for 5 sets

30 air squats

20 strict dips

10 strict chest-to-bar pull-ups
(with vest)

5

Mentality

I love to train scared, so I was really in my element in the lead-up to the 2016 Regionals.

Unlike at the Games, the events for Regionals are announced a few weeks ahead of time, so obviously you practice them beforehand. And I don't mean you do them half-assed at the end of the day. I'd approach them as seriously as if they were the final event at the Games and bury myself trying to get the best score.

Of the seven Regionals workouts in 2016, I was pretty satisfied with six, but there was one I couldn't finish: Strict Nate—10 rounds of 4 strict muscle-ups, 7 strict handstand push-ups, and 12 kettlebell snatches. I did it a few times, and the best I ever got was seven rounds and change. That didn't feel great at first but wasn't a disaster because some workouts are specifically designed to be unbeatable. Then I realized that this wasn't one of them.

Usually, I'd never share any information about my training—you've always got to maintain that edge—but that year I was swapping scores with Alex Anderson, who was competing in a different region. During practice, his Strict Nate score was better than mine, and I watched as other guys posted videos of their attempts on Instagram. It seemed like everyone was finishing but me.

Okay, I tried to reassure myself. *You can upload whatever you want to social media, but all that matters is what happens on the floor.* And, because I was in the third and final region to compete that year, I'd have the advantage of seeing them all attempt Strict Nate before I did.

Six guys finished it in the first week, and seven more the week after. *Yikes,* I told myself. *This is the year you don't qualify. This is the year you don't have what it takes.* I could already hear people talking about why I'd fallen off and how I just didn't have what it took to stand on top of the podium.

So when I finally got to Regionals, it didn't matter that I won the first event. As the countdown started for Nasty Nate, I knew I was about to be embarrassed, so I refused to relent for even a second. No extra-long chalk breaks. No dropping into a squat and catching my breath. If I wanted a shot at the Games that year, I had to drive full speed into the pain cave.

At the same time, I couldn't watch what the other competitors were doing and change my pace to race them. I had to "stay in my lane" and get the best score for me.

I ended up finishing the workout in 18:30—almost 50 percent faster than in practice. It was such an unbelievable improvement that Alex was convinced I'd lied to him. I hadn't. I just tend to do my best when I feel like my back is against the wall.

Well, kind of.

I wish I could say that my mental prep is as straightforward as training scared, but it's more complicated than that. For me to be the best version of myself, I have to simultaneously believe that I'm overrated and invincible, that I'm an impostor on the verge of being humiliated on the competition floor, and that I'm an untouchable Lamborghini in a sea of broken-down hooptiers.

Mentality 101

JOURNAL ENTRY—*15:00*

When it comes to fitness, what do you take for granted? What came naturally to you, what did you pick up faster than the people around you, or what were you already able to do? It can be something as small as already having double-unders or as big as learning a muscle-up in your first month of CrossFit. Before you train your weaknesses, it's helpful to know the strengths that you overlook.

I like to say that the best thing to ever happen to me in CrossFit was losing the 2015 Games. That loss forced me to work hard and take this sport seriously, but there was another event that may have been even more important.

It was during Event Four of the 2013 Regionals, my first sanctioned CrossFit competition. The day before, I'd set the world record in the three-rep overhead squat, but now I was struggling through a workout called The Hundreds: 100 wall-balls, 100 chest-to-bars, 100 pistols, and 100 single-arm snatches. I'd expected to blow through the last movement, but my lungs were screaming, and I got through only 67 snatches. But that's not what my judge wrote down. See, every time you finished 20 reps, you moved forward on the floor and stood on top of the number you had to hit before moving on. So when the time ran out, I was above the number 80, and my judge recorded 87 reps.

When I realized her mistake, I beelined to where the judges were and tapped her on the arm. *What're you doing?* she said, gesturing around here. *We're in the middle of a meeting.* I tried to tell her she'd screwed up my score, but she shook her head and turned around. *No, no, no. The score's good.* But when I said she'd given me 20 reps too many, I got her attention, and they corrected it. At the weekend, I realized that I would've gone to the Games if I'd kept my mouth shut. But thank God I didn't.

I'd done practically nothing to get ready for Regionals, and if I'd been rewarded with a ticket to the Games, I probably would've trained even less and shown up totally unprepared. Then I would've packed it in as soon as I hit an event where I couldn't just impress everyone with my brute strength. I barely rowed 1 kilometer at Regionals without stopping, and on the very first day at the Games, I would've had to row 21,097 meters? Yeah, that would've been a hard pass from me.

It took me years—and a few very public humiliations—to decide that I wanted to be the Fittest on Earth. So what I want you to do right now is evaluate how seriously you want to take this sport. Be honest with yourself. Maybe you don't want to be the absolute best athlete you can be. That's okay. Believe me, I know how much work it takes.

In the last few weeks leading up to the Games, my entire life—and Sammy's—would revolve around my health and safety. I'd stop riding my motorcycle, even just around our neighborhood. I'd refuse to go to the beach in case there was broken glass I could step on. I'd even stop using a steak knife because what if this was the one time in a million that I cut my hand?

So what're your goals? Maybe you want to be number one at your gym but never compete. Maybe you want to get a specific skill, like a ring muscle-up or a bodyweight snatch. Maybe you just like going to the gym every day, breaking a sweat, and hanging out with your buddies, and you'd be happy maintaining where you're at. Those are great goals, and you can always change them as you get more experience, just like I did. So decide what your personal podium is and work toward it.

Where you'll run into problems is if your expectations don't align with the amount of work you're willing to invest, and so many CrossFit athletes assume they've got what it takes to focus on nothing but eating, sleeping, and training. Before you download your 12-week strength plan, meal prep for the next month, and buy every supplement that's advertised to you on Instagram, you have to ask yourself: That thing I hate doing, am I willing to do it every day for a year?

That's what I did with rowing, and then sprinting, then deadlifting, and then swimming, and the list goes on and on. To be a true competitor, you have to accept that you'll always be working most on the thing you like least. No matter how many times you win the Games, there's an endless list of weaknesses to improve—and that should scare you.

Training Scared

JOURNAL ENTRY—*15:00*

What are your weaknesses—not the things that you're currently bad at, but what's most difficult for you to learn? Where are you seeing the lowest ratio of work to reward?

I didn't know it at the time, but my weaknesses became the reason I stayed in the sport. If I'd won the Games the first year I went, I never could've taken CrossFit seriously. *You're telling me I could walk out onto the field, still sluggish from the Chinese food I ate the night before, and beat guys who've trained for this for years?* But once I realized it'd be more difficult than that, I started to truly fall in love.

I started noticing that I was terrified before workouts, which was a new feeling for me. I'd get nervous at weightlifting meets, but it was such a different experience. I'd be alone on the platform for 30 seconds, and either I'd hit the lift or not. I was never struggling to breathe or taking a knee while the other athletes passed me by, leaving me alone on the floor while everyone watched me try to finish the workout. The discomfort in Olympic weightlifting was so different from the discomfort in CrossFit.

That fear is what ultimately attracted me to the sport, like a ledge you know is too high to jump off but can't resist looking over the edge of. I didn't recognize that at the time, but Ben Bergeron, a coach I worked with for a few years, certainly did.

In 2014, I would travel from Vermont to his gym outside Boston, and nearly every time I was there, he had me do the same workout with the same guy. I knew I was fitter than Connor, but he was also six-two, so every time we got to the part where we had to do the burpee pull-ups, he barely had to jump. He could recover during this section, whereas I'd be doing a max effort jump just to start my pull-up. Even when I beat him, it wasn't by much, and I'd leave rattled. *I need to work harder. I need to improve my mobility. I need to find every inch of benefit I can.*

JOURNAL ENTRY—*15:00*

If a film crew were coming to your gym, but they would record you doing only one movement, which one would it be? And which movement would be the last one you'd ever want the world to see? Explore why that is for both. Is it because of the weight you can (or can't) lift? The strengths (or gaps) you have in your technique? Understanding why you're proud of certain exercises can help you identify where your ego may be getting too involved.

The most fundamental part of training scared is that you bury your ego regardless of how much success you had the day before. That's a difficult mindset to get into, but there was a movement that always reminded me not to take myself too seriously: pistol squats.

For years, I listened to the CrossFit commentators speculate about why I grabbed my toe at the bottom of a pistol. They'd say it was to take some of the strain off the hip flexor of my lead leg. But at the elite level, no one's hip flexor burns out from pistols. The commentators were wrong.

Grabbing my toe pulled my torso forward and made it more of a quad-dominant movement. It wasn't faster, but it used less energy, so it was worth doing even though everyone criticized it.

It reminds me of an old joke. A kid's getting teased for how dumb he is, and the bully holds out a dime and nickel and asks him which one he wants. The kid takes a nickel because he says it's the bigger one. Every day, the bully does the same thing to show his friends how dumb this kid is. One day, a father grabs the kid and is like, "You know the dime is more valuable, right?" "Of course I know," says the kid. "But if I prove to him I know the difference, I don't get a nickel every day."

An advantage is only an advantage if no one else is doing it, so that's why I've never corrected the commentators before. Sometimes your training hacks can make you look like a badass, and sometimes they make you look like a newbie.

JOURNAL ENTRY—*15:00*

You wake up the morning of competition and are able to control only one of the following: what you eat for breakfast, the time your event starts, the length of your warm-up, whether the workout is indoors or outdoors, or who else is in your heat. Which one do you choose and why? Where do you need certainty, and where are you able to be a bit more flexible?

I think training scared was also one of the reasons I was able to handle the unknown especially well. I was nervous about how I'd perform eleven months out of the year, so I didn't fall apart when I got to the Games and had no idea what I'd be doing for the next five days.

I remember the other athletes being especially anxious at the 2016 Games. The day before the start of the competition, we were told three things. One, we had to be in the lobby at 3:30 the next morning. Two, if we weren't there on time, the bus would leave without us. Three, to bring a valid ID. That was it, and the rumors started to fly. We were doing the ocean swim before sunrise. We were flying to Vegas for an ultra-marathon. We were being dropped on a mountaintop and told to survive.

The next day, we found out we were going to the airport, and everyone broke off into speculation again. Where could we be going? How long was the flight? Would we be coming back that night?

Moments like these are especially nerve-racking for athletes who like to be in control of everything, which is usually possible when you're training at your home gym. You decide when to wake up, use your favorite barbell, listen to your playlists, and sleep in your own bed. But all that goes out the window at the Games, and the nerves don't just go away after the workout is announced.

Maybe the event will be something familiar, like a one-rep snatch or a Hero workout you've done a thousand times. But it's probably going to be something you've never done before, whether that means an entirely new apparatus, like the Pig flip or the peg-board, or just familiar movements combined in a unique way. At least you get to see some of the athletes do the workout before you if you're in a later heat, but no matter what, you get only one shot at it. So how do you set your pace? When do you take a break? Which way makes the most sense to cycle the barbell?

No one can be 100 percent sure of the answer ahead of time, not even me. But I had an advantage: I never felt totally in control of my training. Up until the last event at the Games, I was always terrified that I'd forgotten something important, like a dream where you realize you never took the final exam in your high school calculus class and you can't graduate from college until you do. So as much as I hated that feeling of training scared for so many years, I know it accounted for half of my success. The other half was doing the exact opposite.

Seeming Invincible

JOURNAL ENTRY—20:00

Brainstorm five ways that you can trigger a mental shift from being nervous to feeling invincible. Is it a song that you listen to only before competition? A mantra you repeat in your head as you warm up? A memory you can recall of a time you felt especially confident? A smell that reminds you of another athletic accomplishment? Even if you aren't naturally confident, you can fake it 'til you make it by developing rituals.

No matter how nervous I was before an event—no matter how hard I was dry heaving in the athlete corral right before my heat was called—I knew that I had to flip a switch the second I walked out onto the floor. From that moment on, I had to seem invincible.

To make this transition possible I almost never posted videos of myself training, not even if I PRed my snatch by 25 pounds. I get why athletes are so active on social media, but you're giving your competitors an endless stream of information about your potential weaknesses. Especially after I won the Games for the first time in 2016, all I wanted the other guys to know about me was that I'd beaten them the last time we'd competed together. If they didn't know anything other than that, their minds would fill in the details using their own doubts and insecurities. Whenever they thought of me, they'd picture my highlight reel, and I would seem unbeatable.

I also never talked shit, not on social media, not in the warm-up area, not in the post-workout interviews. It's not my style to begin with, and I also knew that beating my chest and saying that So-and-So was overrated would only give that guy an ego boost. Even if I did notice what someone was up to during the off-season, or how their top lifts were inching up toward mine, I'd definitely never say so. I didn't want anyone thinking I considered them a threat.

And there was something else I did to maintain my aura of invincibility that was even more extreme, and it almost backfired on me a few times.

JOURNAL ENTRY—*20:00*

Injuries are an inevitable part of being an athlete, so what is your go-to method of coping when you feel a pinch, tweak, or pop? Do you collapse to the ground and call over the coach? Do you take a break, stretch out a bit, then get back to it? Do you overcompensate by doubling down and finishing the workout even faster? Do you tend to assume the worst—that your athletic career is over—or underestimate what's happened and push through?

It didn't matter if I impaled myself with a barbell and was bleeding out on the lifting platform, I would do everything possible to hide an injury from my competitors.

An example that comes to mind is the first day of the 2017 Games. In the warm-up area about 45 minutes before the third event, I was in a pigeon stretch on a box when I heard and felt a pop in my knee. I froze. I looked around. The good news was that no one had noticed. The bad news was that a pop that loud couldn't be a good sign.

I pulled my heel up to my butt a few times. That felt fine. I did a couple air squats. No pain there, either. But then I raised my leg out to the side and shook it, and the only way I can describe its movement was "sloppy," like the joint was only 75 percent connected. What had I done?

The way I saw it, there were three possible outcomes for the next workout. The first was that something in my knee was torn completely, and I'd realize pretty quickly that I'd have to withdraw.

The second was that it was a partial tear, and I'd tear it completely. Again, I'd have to withdraw. The third was that I'd go to the medical staff, and regardless of how bad it really was, they might get spooked and medically withdraw me.

No matter what, a year's worth of effort would be down the drain, so which option would give me the best chance of squeaking through the rest of the Games? Certainly not the personal trainers. So I might as well roll the dice and do the next workout. Odds were that I already needed surgery anyway, so if my knee blew out, my knee blew out.

But if I was going to compete, I had to hide the injury from everyone, even Sammy and O'Keefe, whom I see before and after every event. If I told them what had happened, my biggest fear was that they'd start to treat me differently, which would make me doubt myself.

Miraculously, I was able to finish the workout without snapping my leg in half. In fact, I won it, mainly because my knee was fine as long as it was moving forward or backward, not laterally. Still, I asked my mom, a family physician, to stop by my hotel room later that night. She must have known something was seriously wrong because I never see my family during the Games.

When she got to my room, I told her what had happened, and she told me it was impossible to tear your own ligament stretching. Still, I lay down, and she did a few quick mobility checks. *It looks like you stretched it a bit too much,* she said. *And now there's some residual slack.* What she didn't say—but probably knew from that three-minute exam—was that I'd torn my LCL. I'd find that out afterward, but in the moment I chose to believe her. I knew she was lying, but it was just convincing enough that I could tell myself otherwise. *I only strained my knee. It's fine.*

I'm guessing my mom told my dad, but neither of them said a word about it the rest of the weekend, and neither did I. I was still aware of it, but I didn't let it consume me emotionally, especially as the Games wore on, when it was pretty clear that my knee would hold as long as I didn't pivot on it. So avoiding that movement became just another part of my technique, like making sure I pulled the barbell in toward my body during a snatch.

Even after the Games were over, I didn't broadcast my injury. I didn't want to explain what happened a thousand times over and listen to everyone have an opinion about it. So even though it was the hottest part of the summer, I wore pants over the leg brace for the next three or four months.

Then, the following year, I had to hide another injury.

JOURNAL EXERCISE—20:00

The mental and emotional part of an injury can be way worse than the physical pain, so identify what the most stressful part of your recovery is. Do you constantly worry that you're not healing—or not healing as quickly as you want? Are you consumed by watching your competitors improve while you're stuck on the sidelines? Do you feel guilty for whatever mistake led to your injury (or whatever mistake you imagine led to your injury)?

On the third day of competition at the 2018 Games, I was coming down the cargo net on the obstacle course when I lost my grip.

As I fell toward the ground, I naturally curled up a bit, so when my foot got caught on the net, it yanked my leg straight and pulled my hip flexor. I knew something was wrong but still finished the rest of the event. This time, though, there was no hiding what had happened. Everyone saw me tumble and hit the sand.

One of the Games staff came up and asked what was wrong after I crossed the finish line. I told him nothing, and he knew I was lying and poked me, hoping that I'd wince and he could call over the medical team. He started with the shoulder, which is the part of my body I landed on hardest. Surprisingly, it didn't hurt, and there was no reaction from me. *Please don't touch my hip,* I thought. Then the ribs. Also fine. *Please don't touch my hip.* Then my quad. No pain there, either. He didn't see the bruising up and down my hip flexor and walked away. Like everyone else, he was too distracted by someone else: Pat Vellner.

Vellner also fell off the cargo net, but he took the opposite approach. Instead of playing down the injury, he flagged the medical staff as soon as he finished. Vellner ate it hard off the cargo net, and I didn't blame him for thinking he'd punctured a lung, especially because he was spitting up blood. But here's the thing— when the doctors told him to go to the hospital, he didn't want to go.

This was hard for me to understand. He'd just fallen eight feet and slammed into the ground. What was he hoping the CrossFit medical staff could do in that situation? Was he hoping primarily for reassurance that he was okay? Probably. But most likely they would need to recommend he get tested to make sure he wasn't bleeding internally. And even if they didn't medically pull him from the competition, they were certainly going to watch him more carefully. So why even bother calling the medical team over if you're going to refuse to go to the hospital?

JOURNAL ENTRY—20:00

The next time you go to the doctor, she hands you an envelope and tells you that written inside is your VO$_2$ max. What do you hope the number is and why? Do you want it to be off-the-charts high so you know that you could be smashing workouts if you improved the mental side of training? Or do you want it to be super low—proof that you have an amazing pain tolerance? Or would you prefer something in the middle?

Maintaining that illusion of being invincible—for the other competitors and for myself—was nonnegotiable, and it definitely caused some tension with my coaches. For example, at the beginning of the 2015 season, Ben Bergeron wanted all his athletes to have their blood and sweat analyzed to get a custom diet plan based on their genetics. I told him I wasn't going to look at the results—I was still eating pizza, ribs, and Chinese food from the truck outside the library and had no intention of stopping—but I did it anyway.

A few weeks later, curiosity got the best of me, and I opened the results. All I saw was one graph. It was the standard range of testosterone, and my dot was well below the bottom line. Without reading another word, I closed out the email and sat in front of my computer. There it was. I had low T. So how was I going to win the CrossFit Games?

Throughout that entire season, anytime I felt like I hadn't recovered, or I couldn't hold my splits on the rower, or I wasn't hitting the weights I wanted, that email was in my head. *It's not your fault. You're doing great for someone who has low testosterone. You just don't have the energy to beat the best.* Not even taking second at the Games eliminated those insecurities.

But then I made an offhand comment to my mom about the test results after the season. *There's no chance,* she told me. *You're the hairiest guy out there. You don't have low T.* I pulled up the email for her to read, and she chuckled. What I had seen wasn't my own results. It was the example for how to read the graph.

The lesson was clear: Tests like these had the power to mess with my head. Sometimes that was good. My scores for lactic threshold were about as good as they could be, better than some of the best soccer players in the world. The doctor had compared me with a Lamborghini—amazing power output and terrible gas mileage (hence why I'm so quick to overheat and sweat like the world's ending). That was great to hear, and during the trail run at the 2020 Games, when I needed to put the hammer down and smoke Justin Medeiros in the last half mile, I pictured myself as a Lamborghini.

But that didn't mean my other metrics would be so amazing. That's why I refused to test my VO_2 max, the measure of how much oxygen your body can absorb and use during exercise, no matter how many times Hinshaw asked me to. What if it were good, better than average but lower than my competitors'? How could that not be in the back of my mind during every cardio workout at the Games?

My mindset was such a careful balancing act that I would swerve between thinking I was the greatest and the worst not just over the course of one day, but even during a single workout.

During the 2020 season, I'd practice my Assault Bike intervals in front of a mirror, and sometimes I'd see myself and be disgusted by how weak I looked—face grimacing, shoulders slouched, head tilted down. And that's exactly when I knew I had to go 10 percent harder. Because the only thing that would make me just a little bit less scared was the confidence that I could endure pain better than anyone else.

JOURNAL ENTRY—*15:00*

Before your next five workouts, write down an estimate of your score (either the time or the total number of reps). Afterward, go back and see how accurate your prediction was. Did you tend to overestimate your performance or to sell yourself short? Identifying your mindset in this way can help you determine whether you need to talk yourself up or hold yourself back.

It's obviously difficult to go between these two contradictory mindsets, and if I had to choose only one, I'd train scared.

When I was a teenager, I'd go to the local lake and dive off the cliffs that were thirty-five, forty feet up. What really made it dangerous was that you had to jump between a hole in the rocks in order to make it into the water below—and that water was only about six feet deep. We'd scrape our bellies on the bottom all the time.

I've always been blessed with a lot of natural athleticism and body awareness, so I'd get some cuts and bruises but nothing serious. Then I started listening to my ego. If we were there and some guy threw a backflip, I'd throw a backflip. Then he'd throw a double backflip, so I'd throw a double backflip. Of all the stupid and reckless antics I did as a kid, this was one of the only times that I was attempting stunts that were truly above my abilities. Thankfully, my parents convinced me to tone it down before I smashed my head trying to do a double gainer.

I learned how to control my ego as I've gotten older, but not always. Case in point: At the 2016 Regionals, two days after I won Nasty Nate, the event I couldn't even finish in practice, we did a workout that was essentially 45 thrusters with a few legless rope climbs sprinkled in. I don't think anyone in the world is better than I am at 95-pound thrusters, so on paper, I should've won this workout easily. I didn't get smashed by any means—I took second—but I was so overconfident that I walked during my transitions between the barbell and the rope. There was no fear pushing me forward.

It was a great reminder that, especially in the heat of a workout, when my heart rate was jacked up and my body temperature was starting to spike, I couldn't be fully trusted to decide when to throttle back. In CrossFit, the name of the game is suffering, and there's nothing you can do but lean into it.

Pain Tolerance

JOURNAL ENTRY—20:00

Describe the most painful workout you've ever done, starting with the warm-up. How fresh were you going into it,
and what did you expect it to be like? When did you realize
that you were entering the Pain Cave, and how did your
pace and intensity change? Where in your body did you
feel the discomfort most? Your lungs, which felt like they
were filling up with water? Your quads, which had jolts of
electricity zapped into them? Your forearms, which felt so
swollen you could barely bend your fingers at the knuckles, let alone close your hands? Try to recall the experience as vividly as possible.

Saying you're ready to suffer is easy when you're in the comfort
of the warm-up area. But then you've got a barbell in your hands,
and the weight and friction of it is ripping the skin from your
blisters and covering the fresh pink flesh with chalk, sweat, and
blood. The harder you push, the more oxygen your muscles need,
and the heavier you start to breathe. The force of hyperventilating
causes your capillaries to release fluid, flooding your lungs with
enough liquid to simulate the effects of drowning, and you lose
the ability to focus, recall memories, and even count reps. For up
to a full day after you stop moving, you wheeze, hear your lungs
crackle, and taste iron from the fluid you've coughed up.

No matter how many times you've worked out like this, it's hard to remember exactly how bad it hurts. Thankfully, I learned about pain tolerance from an early age.

Both of my parents were Olympic ice skaters for Canada, and one time they were filming an episode of *Stars on Ice* when my dad accidentally pulled my mom off her feet. They told me that her head hit the ground so hard that the technicians in the sound booth came out to investigate. They thought that the chandelier had fallen from the ceiling.

But even if a skill went so wrong that my mom had to finish her routine with a dislocated shoulder, which happened in Spain, they always played it cool on the ice, which was exactly how level-headed they were with us.

One time I was bounced off a trampoline and landed on my side directly on top of a stump. After I recovered from the wind getting knocked out of me, I started to cry, but my mom took my hand, walked me into the kitchen, quickly checked me out, and set me up on the couch to watch a movie. She was a family physician and knew I wasn't seriously hurt, and seeing her being calm calmed me down, too. The next day, I felt good enough to water-ski.

Because we got limited sympathy, it was inevitable that my brother and I were going to be tough. If we were sick or hurt, there was no doting, except in extreme circumstances, like when my mom basically marched into the OTC and demanded that they X-ray my back.

This approach applies to training for CrossFit, too. If you're halfway through a workout and start to tell yourself that you have to catch your breath, or the pain in your legs is only going to get worse, or there's no way you can get back on the rower, you're sunk. So recognize that you're afraid of discomfort, and spend this time with your journal investigating why.

Dealing with Obstacles

JOURNAL ENTRY—*20:00*

Describe the three most embarrassing moments you've had in your athletic career.

In 2014, a girl from my gym asked if I wanted to go with her to take the L-1 class, the certification you need to become a CrossFit coach. I wanted to impress her, so I said yes, and I still don't know what I did to upset the head coach, but he took any opportunity to humiliate me in front of the rest of the group.

We were all in a circle practicing an overhead squat, and he yelled out that my knees tracked too far forward. I nodded my head but didn't change my technique. I'd spent a decade learning how to do this lift correctly, along with some help from Team USA. So the coach stopped the class and escorted me to the edge of the class. *I want you to put your toes against the wall,* he told me as everyone else watched.

Hey man, I know what you're doing here, and I don't appreciate it, I told him. He slapped me on the back. *Ah, man, we're all friends here,* he said. I put my toes against the wall, squatted down, hit my knees, and fell onto my ass. Everyone chuckled. *It doesn't matter how much weight you can do*, he said. *You can't build off your foundation if you don't have proper technique.*

At the end of class, I got to have my revenge. Everyone did the same workout of 21–15–9 of thrusters and burpees, and the coach went out of his way to remind us that his athlete had the world record for it. He'd done it in 3:30, so I decided to sell my soul to beat that time. As soon as the coach saw how fast I was going, he came over to ref me like we were at Regionals, but I knew my form was perfect. *Bro, it's thrusters and burpees. You really think you're going to no-rep me on this?* I finished in three minutes flat. Instead of congratulating me, he just walked away.

I never learned the guy's name, but he had some very distinct tattoos on his arms, so I recognized him the second I saw him in the warm-up area at the 2014 Games. I'd just finished the one-rep max overhead squat. I stared at him, but he never made eye contact, probably because he didn't want to acknowledge what had just happened: I'd won it with 377 pounds.

That experience taught me that success is the best revenge, which is how I coped with some other obstacles in my career.

JOURNAL ENTRY—*15:00*

For your next three workouts, find someone to judge you and make sure you're always hitting the movement standard. Then record the times you were no-repped and why.

All sports have a certain degree of subjectivity, which is especially true in CrossFit, where you have to meet a movement standard, like squatting below parallel or getting your chin above the bar on a pull-up. Games athletes definitely don't make judging easy because we're usually cranking out reps as fast as we can. For example, when we did Mary in 2019, I ended up with 675 reps, about one every 1.75 seconds.

In competition, I was also trying to do as little work as possible, so there was room for people to reasonably disagree over my judge's call. But here's the thing: There's no point in disagreeing.

The rule in CrossFit is that the judge's decision is final, and no amount of screaming and shouting is going to change their mind. It's only going to waste your time. If you're caught in that situation, you have to take a deep breath, suck it up, and keep going.

To make sure you avoid that situation, always practice your movements using the Games standard. That way, you don't have to change a thing during competition. Also, go over the standard with your judge beforehand. What they've been taught is a general rule—like squat below parallel—but that may look different on your body than on someone else's. If you both know exactly what they're looking for and how that feels, there shouldn't be any confusion during the workout.

If you do get no-repped, you may want to ask the judge why, but don't expect a satisfying answer because judges aren't required to explain their reasoning. If it keeps happening, you may have to exaggerate the movement even though it's a waste of your time and energy.

At Regionals in 2016, I was one round into a three-rounder

of deadlifts, GHDs, and a run when a judge came up to me and said that I wasn't allowed to wear grips. I was fuming because they never mentioned that rule during the briefing, and five others guys in my heat were wearing them. *Go make Paul Tremblay take his off,* I told the judge *No,* he said. *Just you.*

The grips saved me time by not having to chalk for the deadlift, but I ripped them off and kept going—until the third round. That's when the same judge came up to me, handed me my grips, and said I could put them on. No explanation for why.

If you've ever worn grips, you know that they're a pain in the ass to put on. You have to slide your fingers through the eyelets and then thread the Velcro through the wrist strap, so getting them onto my hands would've taken longer than just chalking my hands. I threw them to the side.

I ended up finishing the workout in sixth, three places lower than I'd hoped for, but I didn't file a rebuttal. It would've been impossible to know how many seconds I lost, and I had a big enough lead that year that I didn't think it'd drop me out of contention for the Games.

That experience was a good reminder that you can't 100 percent count on anything, not even something as minor as grips. What if CrossFit got into a disagreement with its grip sponsor and then decided that no one could wear grips during the next competition? That wouldn't be the craziest thing to happen in the sport, and leading up to the Games I would run tons of these kinds of scenarios and what-ifs. And then train for them. Nothing was off the table and nothing was too far-fetched.

Hard Work Pays Off

JOURNAL ENTRY—_20:00_

Ask a friend (or an enemy) to no-rep you once during your next workout, even if you're following the movement standards perfectly. Then record how you reacted to the setback.

At the 2019 Games, I didn't realize when the weight fell out of my ruck bag at the beginning of Day 2. I was already 25 minutes into the run, so even though I felt something hit my foot as I rounded the last turn before entering the stadium, nothing was there when I looked back. I kept going, finished the last little bit, and threw my ruck in the pile that had formed on the AstroTurf.

This was a gnarly workout, especially because of the friction from the ruck rubbing against your back. Some of the athletes finished covered in blood, and even though I wasn't in that bad of shape, I was definitely ready to take an ice bath before the next event. But a judge stopped me as I was walking off the field and asked for my bag. Sometimes the equipment they give us has our names stitched into it, like the weighted vest, but all the rucks were unmarked and identical, so I picked a random one off the pile, handed it to the judge, and walked away. Another event done, or so I thought.

A little bit later, I was getting body work done when a CrossFit official found me and said I'd been penalized a full minute. My jaw dropped. The bag fell out 28 seconds before I crossed the finish line, so why wasn't the penalty 28 seconds? _Well,_ he said.

We doubled it and rounded up. There was nothing I could do. The decision was final, so I got back to my body work.

That didn't mean the ordeal was over. Later in the day, I realized that the director of the Games had posted a clip of what had happened to social media, and everybody was more than happy to call me a cheater. *Look at him turn around,* they said. *He knew what he was doing.* Going into a mental spiral would've hurt me much more than the original penalty, so I put away my phone and focused on the upcoming events.

It wasn't easy to move on, which is why you need to practice. Believe me, one no-rep may not sound like a big deal before the workout, but when you're at the edge of the Pain Cave or think you're about to finish, it can feel like the end of the world.

Developing Curiosity

JOURNAL ENTRY—*30:00*

Write down everything you remember about the person closest to you during your last workout. What were they wearing? How much weight was on their bar? Did they finish before or after you? Scale or do the workout Rx? Collapse onto the ground afterward or pace around trying to catch their breath?

If you want to be a great athlete, you have to be curious, especially about your own body. That's why I love EMOMs so much. You know the workload you have to complete and the time to get it done, so there's no holding back. Either you finish or you don't, and I've done things I truly didn't think I was capable of, like 40 minutes of a 200-meter row (minute 1), 200-meter SkiErg (minute 2), 200-meter Assault Bike (minute 3), and 50 double-unders (minute 4).

But if you want to be an elite athlete, you also have to be curious about the circumstances you'll compete in. As soon as it was announced that the Games were moving from California to Madison, Wisconsin, I booked a flight out there and started to explore. The city's pretty close to a few parks, so I visited them all and asked what kinds of events they hosted: hikes? Trail runs? Maybe rock climbing?

I also knew that Madison was famous for triathlons, so I started scoping potential routes that the course could take. When it came to the run, where were the closest hills, and was there a nearby stadium, which would mean stair runs? Because there's always a swim event at the Games, I checked out the lakes in the center of downtown. Where could we enter the water from? How big did the waves get? Would it be clear enough for me to see if my goggles slipped off?

I also looked at another great source of information: the sponsors' page. As soon as a company signs with CrossFit, it's usually written into the contract that their logo has to appear on the site. So in the lead-up to the 2020 Games, I saw Assault Fitness and knew we'd be on their runners, along with GORUCK (a ruck race), and 5.11 (weighted vests). Trek Bikes is based in Wisconsin, so I was pretty confident we'd be biking. This didn't mean I had a full list of the events. Far from it. Just because we were on a Trek bike didn't tell me if it was a 100-meter sprint or a 100-mile ride. But it certainly gave me time to practice everything—and to get used to the equipment.

If you're just looking to work out and have a good time, there isn't really a difference between an AssaultRunner and a True-Form Runner. But if you've got ambitions to compete, these details matter. Each machine has its own feel, so I made sure to practice with what we were going to be competing on. For example, during the 2019 season we knew that every competition had already signed deals with Assault, so Rogue would only have one chance to showcase its own stationary bike during the Rogue Invitational. They were absolutely going to have us use it during that competition—and make sure it was on camera for as long as possible.

Tia and I got the Echo Bike and started to experiment. How many calories could we get in a minute? Did it matter if we started pedaling when the screen was on or off? Did it help to ramp up and then come back down, or to hold the same intensity the entire time?

Even on movements I'd done thousands of times, I tested as many variations as possible. What if I used different grips? Or wore sweatpants instead of shorts? With or without gloves? Wearing a shirt or not? With a hairy chest or shaved?

But no matter how much you know about the venue or the equipment, nothing will ever be as important as your situational awareness. A guy may have a reputation for going out hot and imploding halfway through, but maybe this is the one workout where he learned to pace and is only getting faster with each round. Or maybe you're far enough ahead of your competitors that you can throttle back a bit and start to recover for the next event.

That was where I was during the first event of Phase Two of the 2020 Games, when we had to do five rounds of muscle-ups and shoulder-to-overheads. I was consistently faster than the other four guys and built up a decent lead by doing virtually all the jerks unbroken. But they were heavy (235 pounds) and I misjudged the last one, pressed the barbell halfway above my head, stalled out, and ended up dropping it behind me.

If you were watching the broadcast, you would've thought I'd just lost the entire competition. *A rare no-rep from Mat Fraser,* one of the commentators said. *That was a failure rep,* said another. *That wasn't a misstep.* It's unnerving anytime you get a no-rep, but I wasn't particularly rattled. I was tracking where the second-place guy was, so I knew I had enough time to take a breath, reset, and try again. I won that workout by about ten seconds.

The Optimum Conditions

JOURNAL ENTRY—*30:00*

For the next week, estimate and then measure your body temperature at the end of every workout and then again after a five-minute cold shower.

At the Games, the conditions are never going to be what you'd prefer, so you have to do the best you can.

For me, that meant doing everything I could to stay cool.

Thankfully, the leader's jersey at the Games is white—but for the first few years, I'd be shirtless the entire time I competed. Slowly, I realized that wasn't the smartest choice and experimented with other options. Would I be cooler if I stayed covered (especially my head)? Could I protect my shoulders so they wouldn't get sunburned, which made every shoulder-to-overhead that much more painful? And if I did take off my shirt, was it close enough that I could put it on again if I overheated? These decisions seemed tiny until I was seeing stars and about to collapse from heat exhaustion.

Sometimes I could also stay cool by lucking out and finding shade during a workout, but that only helped so much. There was heat from the air convecting around me, not to mention the radiation coming from the ground. In fact, the rubber below AstroTurf can be so much hotter that you literally feel the difference when you're at the bottom of a burpee.

Even if I didn't notice the heat when I finished a workout, I'd dunk my head in the watercooler immediately afterward. That was often the treat that I'd promise myself halfway through the event, and it was a great way to start cooling down before I could find an ice bath. Your core temperature can stay elevated for hours after you finish your last workout, and if I wanted to sleep well, I had to get cool.

Especially if you tend to train at night, play around with a cool shower post-workout, which may help you fall and stay asleep. Also, make sure your bedroom is cold. Our house is always at 67, 68 degrees, the coldest the AC will go, and I'd like my bedroom to be even colder if possible—anything to help me sleep better.

JOURNAL ENTRY— *20:00*

Every morning, record your sleep quality and length. Even if you have a fitness tracker that monitors your sleep, nothing beats your own self-evaluation.

Many athletes overlook sleep, but it was my number one recovery and rehab tool. Especially in season, I aimed for ten hours every night (though I usually ended up with around nine). That meant everything that emitted blue light (the TV, my phone, a computer) was off by 10 p.m. and I was making a cup of dream, the CBD supplement I used for sleeping. Then Sammy and I played a card game, or I read in dim lighting until I felt tired.

I also made sure my sleeping conditions were perfect. We hung up blackout curtains so our bedroom was totally dark, and I bought a white noise machine and a dawn simulator, basically a giant lightbulb next to our bed that would use light to put me to sleep at night and wake me in the morning. A cooling pad on our mattress would help me get my core temperature down, and as much as I love Sammy, I'd also kick her out of the bed during competition. If she tossed and turned or had to go to the bathroom, it'd throw off my entire night.

During the Games, I'd sleep every chance I got—as late as I could in the morning and then between every event. I also tried to seclude myself as much as possible. Some of the other athletes get a rush from meeting with the fans or watching the earlier heats, but I always thought that was overstimulating, so I'd go back to my hotel room instead of hanging around. In fact, alone time was so important to me that Sammy would rent a house with her family and mine so I could decompress whenever I needed it.

I'm more of a night person, so after the Games my strict bedtime would go out the window. I'd start a series at 11 p.m. and stay up all night to finish it, and sometimes I'd wake up early just because I was so excited not to do anything that day. But most of you don't need help staying up late. You need better discipline going to bed. So set a fixed wake-up time, limit your midday naps, and develop a consistent nighttime routine that includes 30 minutes to wind down, dim lights, and no electronics.

Learning to Love the Rules

JOURNAL ENTRY— *25:00*

Write down every movement standard you can think of for the following exercises: overhead squat, clean and jerk, handstand push-up, American kettlebell swing. Then go look them up. Which ones did you miss? Which ones did you think were requirements but are just good technique? Even if you consistently move well, you've got to know what the rules are if you want to be able to bend them at an elite level.

In order to be successful, you also have to be obsessed with the rules, which is a lesson I learned in middle school when I joined the football team. I expected that someone would eventually explain the game to me. They didn't. Instead, they gave us a huge book of plays and expected us to learn them all. I know now that all the plays are variations on a few basic patterns, but at the time I was totally overwhelmed.

It was the same story with wrestling. There were three big wrestling families in my town, and all those guys had practiced the moves from birth. So when I tried it in middle school, I just got fleeced at the first practice and never went back. It wasn't until I was at the Olympic Training Center and saw the wrestling team train that I realized I might've been decent at it, and I regret letting my embarrassment keep me from going back.

That was why I was so committed to knowing the rules in CrossFit—even when they were unclear. For example, at the end of one of the workouts at the 2016 Games, we had to use a rope to drag a sled across the finish line. There was a box drawn on the floor for us to stand in, and before the event, someone asked what would happen if you stepped outside it. *Don't do that*, they told us. Okay, but what if someone did? *Just don't.*

People realized pretty quickly that it was easier to pull the sled if they leaned all the way back and started to step outside the box. Because there was no clear rule or penalty, all the judges did was keep issuing warnings, and all you had to do was ignore those and keep leaning back.

Almost the same thing happened the next year with the Assault Banger. After 40 calories on the Assault Bike, we had to use a hammer to smash a banger down a 20-foot track. From the second I saw the event, it was obvious that you could hook the hammer on the banger and pull it along the track, so I asked if that'd earn a penalty. Exactly the same response as the year before: *Don't do that*. The guy who won that event smashed and dragged the hammer so badly that they had to replace it for the guy in the next heat.

I was always looking for tiny loopholes in the rules, but I made sure to check that they were legal—just not in front of everyone else. If I thought of a technique that would be faster or easier for a certain movement, I'd wait until the briefing was over, pretend like I'd forgotten to ask my question, and go find the head judge and confirm with him. It didn't matter how small the hack was— like pronating my grip if we had to do double-unders with a heavy rope—I never wanted to give that information away for free. You'd be shocked how many athletes broadcast to everyone a strategy that half of us would never have thought of.

Your Big "Why"

JOURNAL ENTRY—*30:00*

What's your side hustle? If you're thinking of becoming a competitive CrossFit athlete, how are you going to afford the meals, supplements, equipment, and plane tickets out to the Games, all while you're training four to five hours a day? For most people, the only option is a full-time job (probably coaching), but is there another way you can make it work? Is there some skill that you can capitalize on, even if it's not how you want to spend the rest of your life?

Hard Work Pays Off

When your body's doing everything it can to shut you down, it also helps to have a reward in mind for when you finish—and the more primal the better. When I was still living in New England, what got me through a decent number of workouts was the thought of walking outside (crawling if I had to) and face-planting directly into a snowbank. That's how I would ignore the heat pressing against my head and the puddles of sweat forming underneath the Assault Bike.

But at some point, the suffering becomes so intense that there's no treat satisfying enough to get you through it—no snowbank, slice of cheesecake, or day on the lake with friends. And that's when you need your bigger why.

Originally, mine was earning enough pocket money so I wouldn't be dependent on my parents. But then, after my junior year of college in 2014, I got an internship with an aerospace company, which was a dream job for a mechanical engineering major. I mean, this company literally built rockets, but I couldn't have been more unhappy.

This was the kind of place where people said to one another, with all seriousness, *It looks like somebody has a case of the Mondays.* Everything was gray—the carpet, the walls, my cubicle—and I had to wear a button-down shirt and slacks every day. Thank God my boss was also a CrossFit athlete and understood when I asked to take off a week to go to the Games that year, but from just those few months of corporate life, I knew that a desk job wasn't for me.

Still, I didn't dream of dropping out of school. My mom got her medical degree as her skating career was winding down, and

I saw all the opportunities that gave her. Plus, my parents were pretty insistent that education be my number one priority. So I was shocked when they suggested I take a semester off from the University of Vermont and pursue CrossFit full-time. In 2015, CrossFit definitely wasn't what it is now. Nike and Rogue and a very few other big players were sponsors, but I don't know if anybody was making their living just off competitions.

At that point, I was still planning on going back to the oil fields in Alberta after I graduated. All you needed to get a job there was a driver's license and a clean record. You could make a ton of money doing work most other people couldn't stomach, and you'd work your ass off for four days on and then get four days of vacation. That was hard work paying off in action.

So as happy as I was that my parents thought I could make something of myself in CrossFit, I stayed in my last few months of school. I ended up with a double major that I may never use, but seeing another potential career path helped me fully commit to the sport. No matter what happened, there was a fallback plan waiting for me, even if it did give me a case of the Mondays.

JOURNAL ENTRY—*30:00*

Make a bet on yourself. It doesn't have to be with money, and it doesn't have to be related to fitness, but set a goal that you want to accomplish within the next year and set aside something of value. Even if no one else believes in you, there's a huge psychological shift that happens when you prove that you believe in yourself.

Once I decided to commit myself entirely to CrossFit, I bet on myself from the very beginning. Because I was an unproven athlete, sponsors didn't want to pay me very much. But they were willing to double my salary if I won the Games, and to double it again if I won the next year, and again, and again. Even if they thought I could win once, no one believed that anyone would ever be the champion five times in a row, so they were happy to pay me less in the moment in exchange for higher performance bonuses in the future.

By the end of my career, people assumed that I was killing myself all season for the $300,000 check from winning the Games. Don't get me wrong. That's a ton of money and about $299,000 more than I ever thought I'd make when I first started competing in CrossFit. However, it's less when you consider all the time and focus required to get there, and how short your career is in this sport. But because of how I structured my contracts, I gave myself something that I never dreamed of having at thirty: financial freedom.

So there are the ways that I got hyped before an event—picturing myself on the podium, seeing my competitors nervously sway from side to side, hearing the song that Sammy told the DJ to play as I walk out onto the floor. But there's a big difference between what gets your adrenaline pumping in the warm-up area and what's able to carry you through the last 15 percent of the event, when your muscles are failing and you feel like your lungs are collapsing. You're too exhausted to even hear the music playing, and that's when you need your bigger why.

I felt that moment most intensely on the last event at the 2019 Games. If I were to do that workout today, I wouldn't do a single touch-and-go snatch at the end of the workout, after I've already done 30 clean and jerks and 30 muscle-ups. But at the time it didn't matter how much pain I was in. I knew it was going to end after three minutes, and waiting for me at the finish line was the largest check I'd ever gotten. That meant that Sammy and I could both be stay-at-home parents if we wanted to and live in our dream home in Vermont. So if I'd had to do all 30 snatches unbroken, I would've collapsed trying.

How can you structure your life so that your motivation is much bigger than a feeling, that it's an end goal that you can access even in the fog of a near blackout?

6

Recovery

By the end of the 2019 Games, I was ready to finish the final event, leave my shoes on the competition floor, and announce my retirement from CrossFit.

Like at the end of every season, I was burned out. My body hurt in a million different ways, and after an especially stressful weekend of competition, I couldn't imagine doing it all again: day after day of selling my soul to the Assault Bike, running up mountains, drowning in the pool, and brushing up against heat stroke for months on end.

Plus, with the 2019 victory I'd done what everyone had always told me was impossible: won four CrossFit Games consecutively. I was undeniably the best in the sport, and at the time that seemed like enough. But then I did what I always do after the season ends. I took a vacation. Sammy and I drove to a lake where we wouldn't see anyone for days, and in between doing nothing I'd eat a cheesecake for breakfast and a plate of cookies for lunch. I was slowly and eagerly becoming my off-season alter ego: Fat Mat.

I still said that I was done with the sport—at least that's what

I told Shane and Tia when they called me—but I think they knew that wasn't necessarily true, and so did I. It was just part of my recovery process, a way to decompress from the pressure and stress of training before deciding to do it all over again. And it worked (at least for one more go).

After about a month, I got sick of eating until my stomach hurt, lounging around on my phone all day, and even staying up all night to binge *The Office*. So I gradually went back to the gym, sometimes to work out, and sometimes just to stop in, say hi to friends, and maybe hit a couple sets of bench press if I felt like it. There'd be days where I felt excited to work out up to the moment I stepped in the gym. Then, for whatever reason, I'd lose motivation and walk back out the door, something I wouldn't dream of doing during the season.

Easing myself back into training worked. I was hungry to be fit again by October, and that's when I'd start to go through old workouts. Even though I was comparing Fat Mat to Cross-Fit Games Mat, I'd still have the same reaction every day: "Oh no, I lost it." My lifting numbers were garbage. I couldn't pull the same pace on the Assault Bike. I didn't even try to get in the pool and swim intervals. After an off-season of not caring, I'd become scared again—and that's how I knew I was ready for another year of training.

This mental reset is one of the most important ways I recover, but I've also had to learn to recover from physical exhaustion, bad decisions, and even unfair no-reps. That resiliency is fundamental to my success because, especially in CrossFit, you can judge an athlete by how well they recover.

Recovery 101

JOURNAL ENTRY—7 Days

Record every time you drink water—not a protein shake or Gatorade—and how much you drank.

A few months into CrossFit, I learned about recovery the hard way. I was doing the 2013 CrossFit Open, but because of my school schedule, I couldn't go to the gym between the fourth and fifth week. I was at the library almost the entire time, and whenever I got hungry, I ate what was most convenient. I wasn't sleeping, I wasn't hydrating, and I wasn't exercising more than walking up the stairs to my favorite spot in the library.

So, boy, did I feel bad during that fifth and final workout: four minutes to do 15 sets of 100-pound thrusters and 15 chest-to-bars. That isn't a lot of work by itself, but if you finished three rounds before the clock ran out, you got four more minutes to do another three rounds. And if you finished three more rounds, you got four more minutes, and so on.

I could scream through this workout because the thrusters were so light for me. So I kept getting more rounds, and I kept murdering my quads in the process. The next day, I was peeing brown.

This actually didn't seem like that big of a deal at first because I'd peed brown a few times before when I was Olympic lifting. I'd freaked out but eventually realized that it never lasted more than a few hours.

I also felt like I had strep throat, which wasn't a new feeling, either. Before I got my tonsils out at nineteen, I had strep two or three times a year, so I was familiar with the headaches, fatigue, and muscle soreness. I didn't have my tonsils anymore, but especially with the stress of finals, I figured I'd just caught a cold at the end of the Vermont winter.

But then a few months later I took the L-1 course and learned about rhabdomyolysis, what happens when you strain your muscles so hard that their fibers break down and get absorbed into the bloodstream, which can be lethal.

In class that day, we went over the most common causes of rhabdo in CrossFit athletes: bad diet, lack of sleep, not training for a long time and then destroying yourself in a workout. Check, check, check. And then we went over the symptoms: brown piss, fatigue, feeling like you got hit by an NFL linebacker. Check, check, check again.

I was lucky that I was so lazy back then. If I'd kept pushing my body after that Open workout, I could've ended up in the hospital. But even after learning about rhabdo, it took me years to learn how to properly care for myself.

The absolute bare minimum is staying hydrated. Unlike meal prep or mobilization drills, it doesn't require any extra time or foresight, so have a water bottle with you at all times. Then you can graduate to the next step of recovery: listening to what your body is telling you.

JOURNAL ENTRY—3 Days

Write down how you're feeling at least four times a day (say, 9 a.m., noon, 3 p.m., 6 p.m.). What's your energy level and mood? Do you feel stiff, sore, or tight anywhere?

I don't care what your wearable fitness tracker says. If you're feeling like you're at 60 percent, it isn't the right day to max your back squat or retest Fran. This can be a hard truth to swallow, particularly if you're doing someone else's programming. I know because I've ignored this advice over and over.

Even after I broke my back overtraining at the OTC—and my doctor told me I was lucky that I'd be able to run again, let alone keep Olympic lifting—I was committed to pushing through any injury.

A few weeks before the 2014 Games, I was having chest pain that was getting progressively worse. Around 2:30 in the morning on the day I was supposed to do a sprint triathlon, I woke up my mom and told her that I couldn't sleep. In fact, I hadn't really slept for the past three nights and couldn't even take a full breath.

She calmed me down a bit, and I was feeling better around 5:30 a.m., so I decided to do the race anyway. It started with a 750-meter swim in Lake Champlain (no wetsuit), then a 12-mile bike ride (I was the only guy on a mountain bike, which I'd borrowed from a friend), and finished with a 5K run. Afterward I was exhausted, but when I lay down to nap I had chest pain, so my mom took me to the ER.

It turns out that the outside lining of my heart was inflamed (pericarditis), so I was pretty lucky that all I'd lost was a few nights of sleep. But not every signal to slow down is as obvious as this one, and it's easy to ignore a tiny pain until it becomes something more serious than that.

So start developing your body awareness now. It'll be inconvenient at first because you'll have to go out of your way to check in with how you're feeling, but gradually it becomes second nature. Then you'll be better equipped to distinguish between discomfort that you can train through and pain that you should stop and address.

JOURNAL ENTRY—*20:00*

The standard active recovery exercise is 20 minutes of light rowing, but this part of your training can be a bit more flexible than the rest. So brainstorm other ways that you can get blood flowing, ways that feel exciting and not like a chore. Maybe that means jogging a few laps around your favorite park, an easy set of stairs at the local football stadium, or a yoga class.

When it comes to recovery, there are so many factors at play—your diet, sleep, stress levels, daily activity—that it's impossible to predict exactly how you'll feel on any given day. In fact, you could do the same workout two different times. The first leaves you feeling fine, and after the second you're so sore that you have to brace yourself against the wall just to squat down to the toilet seat.

When you're in that much pain, you may want to lie on the couch all day. But you've got to get up and do some light exercise in order to circulate your blood, clear some of the lactic acid out, and reduce the soreness. But the key word here is "light," light enough that you can hold a conversation while you do it.

If light cardio on your own isn't your thing, you can also go into the gym and take it easy. Doing the workout scaled (or extra scaled) is a great way to maintain your routine—but that's easier said than done, especially if you tend to get competitive. So if you feel like you always have to give 100 percent in front of your buddies, definitely try a workout at 60 percent and practice prioritizing your recovery, not your ego.

Regardless of the active recovery you choose, you should feel better by the end of it—warmer, more flexible, less sore. If you don't, that's likely a sign that you've overdone it and need another day (or two) before you're back in fighting shape.

JOURNAL ENTRY—7 Days

Record your body temperature immediately after your workout and then four hours later. You may be surprised how slowly your body cools off.

The other fundamental of recovery is to get your core temperature down after every workout, especially if you're hoping to work out again that day.

The first time I got severe heatstroke during a workout, I had no idea what was wrong with my body. It was Murph at the

2015 Games. The conditions were disgusting—the middle of the afternoon during the summer in California, where the only place hotter than the road was the AstroTurf field.

What I remember most is feeling like the skin on my head had shrunk, like someone had put my head in a microwave and was squeezing it as hard as they could. By the end of it, I was dizzy, seeing stars, and feeling tired—not tired like, *My muscles are sore and I wish this were over.* Tired like, *I could lie down right here on the road and take a nap.* I wondered how long I could curl up on the floor without losing my position. Twenty, maybe 30 seconds? It was absolutely demented thinking, but the heat addles your brain.

Somehow I was able to push through it in 2015 and take second place in Murph, but lots of competitors were destroyed. Kara Saunders fully blacked out on the final mile, and Annie Thorisdottir collapsed on the finish line and ultimately had to withdraw from the Games. The next time we did Murph, the commentators couldn't stop saying that we'd all prepared so much better, and that's why our times were faster. Yeah, that was part of it, but that year it was in the morning and with shade on the field, so it was a totally different event.

Physical Recovery

JOURNAL ENTRY—20:00

Make a list of all your chronic aches, pains, and injuries, along with a ranking of how severe they are.

Injuries are an inevitable part of being an athlete, especially at the elite level. They're going to be frustrating, exhausting, and always longer than you want, but remember this: No one is responsible for your recovery more than you.

After I broke my back, I learned that lesson a few times at the OTC. There was a new crop of trainers there practically every week, and one of them suggested that I get a cortisone injection. Now I know that that would've probably been the worst thing to do. It would've numbed the injury, allowing me to lift heavy and probably break my back permanently. But at the time I was clueless. I thought it was odd that he was going to stick a needle into my spine just as casually as he'd tape an ankle, but he told me it would make me feel better and I could keep lifting, so why would I say no?

Even better, he could do it right then, so I sat on the physical therapy table while he went into the back to grab what he needed. Out of pure coincidence, the head doctor walked past me while I was waiting and asked me how I was doing. I told him what was about to happen, and he started fuming.

When the trainer came back with his syringe, the doctor told him to pack his bags. He couldn't work at the OTC anymore. I felt fortunate that the boss was watching out for me, and I trusted that he was a great doctor. But even that didn't mean I got the care I needed.

It was still weeks before anyone thought to X-ray my back, and that was only after my mom insisted on it. So even if you go to the best specialists and get third and fourth opinions, you're going to suffer the consequences of your decisions, not them.

JOURNAL ENTRY—20:00

Whichever injury you rated as the most painful, research
ways to rehab it and give yourself a two-week recovery
plan.

Ten weeks out from the second phase of the 2020 Games, I
braced myself for a heavy back squat, heard a pop, and felt a sensation like Velcro being torn apart. I was no stranger to weird pop-
ping sounds coming from my back, so I figured that the damage
was already done and did two reps before dumping the barbell
behind me. Over the next few days, my back got so bad that it
hurt whether I was moving, standing still, or lying down, and I had
to pull out of the Rogue Invitational (though I obviously didn't tell
anyone the real reason why).

Two weeks later, I saw a doctor in Cookeville, where I was
living at the time, and he said the scans didn't show any breaks or
dislocations, but he was pretty sure it was a rib injury. That was my
worst fear—that the rib had popped out and torn all the stabilizing
muscles around it. How could I recover from something like that
with only two months until the Games?

The doctor suggested a platelet-rich plasma (PRP) injection,
in which he would draw my blood, harvest the plasma, then inject
it into my spine, back, and ribs. I was in a tough spot, so I was
willing to try anything, but afterward I felt the same, maybe a little
worse considering that it was $1,850 a session, none of which was
covered by insurance.

Not only that, but I'd also need to come back three to four

more times over the next eight weeks, meaning I wouldn't fully recover until basically the moment before I had to leave for California to compete. I was still in so much pain that I could barely sleep, let alone train at the intensity I'd need, so even if I did trust this doctor—which I absolutely didn't—my season would be over, anyway.

On the ride home from that first appointment, I called Alex Guerrero, the body work specialist for Tom Brady. We'd met a few years earlier, and I told him what had happened and why I thought I'd dislocated my rib. *It's not a rib injury,* he told me. He hadn't even seen me in person, let alone done any tests, so how could he be so sure? *Well, does it hurt when you breathe?* I said no and basically invited myself to Florida, where his practice is.

We landed the next day and went straight to see Alex. Just from my description over the phone, he was pretty sure that this was the same injury he'd seen dozens of times with NFL linemen. The problem was my quadratus lumborum, which is a muscle that's so deep in your back that it was easier for him to reach it through my abs. So he'd press his hand underneath a rib, move an organ out of the way, and push until he found my psoas, which he'd grab like it was a damn handrail! Then he'd tell me to pump my knees back and forth while I tried not to scream or cry or punch him in the face.

After barely a half hour of work, he told me that we were going to go squat. *Yeah, right,* I thought. I hadn't done 135 pounds since the injury, but that day I maxed out at more than 400. I was as relieved as I was surprised, especially when Alex said I'd be back to normal within three to five days (I booked six just to be safe).

From then on, Alex would work on Tom Brady until 2 or 3 p.m. and then manhandle my psoas until I thought I'd pass out. He also taught Sammy and O'Keefe how to do it, too, though my psoas was usually so tight that Sammy's fingers would bend backward whenever she tried to dig in there.

When we flew back to Tennessee, I wasn't completely back to normal, and one of Alex's trainers flew out to see me every two weeks until we left for the Games. It never got any less painful, especially when he was digging into my psoas while I rowed. But it worked. My back was never an issue at the Games.

So before you shell out $10,000 for PRP injections or some other expensive procedure, do your homework. A few years back I felt something pinching my hip flexor every time I went below parallel, so I reached out to a movement account I follow on Instagram and told them my symptoms. They responded with a personalized protocol, and two minutes into the first exercise, the pain was gone.

All I had to do was use a band to pull my leg out from my hip joint, and that extra millimeter of space was enough to prevent the pinching. Now, I'm not recommending using Google to supplant medical advice, but it's up to you to be informed about possible treatments and to know what to ask your doctor about, especially if you're about to shell out thousands to have your plasma harvested.

Recovery Mentality

JOURNAL ENTRY— $25{:}00$

It's critical to set aside time to recover mentally and physically, but you can get derailed if you leave something to chance, so plan out your next rest day. Where will you go, what will you eat, and what will your activities be? What will you need to bring (sunscreen, water bottle, meal plans) to make sure you're able to fully recover?

It's easy to believe that recovery means no rules. It's your day off from the gym, so you should enjoy it, right? Maybe by spending the day out on a lake with your friends and getting tossed in an inner tube behind the boat?

Unfortunately, you can't be that chill. Your recovery has to be just as intentional as your workouts, because you're trying to create the ideal conditions for your body and mind. Of course it took me a while to completely embrace this idea. After I broke my back, the doctors told me I could still lift weights as long as I wasn't putting pressure on my spine, so I did bench press and bicep curls and a thousand other things that didn't directly involve my back, but which I definitely knew weren't helping. Gradually, though, I realized the importance of recovery and how you have to follow the spirit of the rule.

Take the day out at the lake: Even ignoring the tubing and how risky it could be (a tweaked shoulder, a bruised knee), the whole day is going to drain your energy. You're out in the sun for hours, you probably aren't drinking enough water, and you're more likely to eat whatever food is being passed around the boat. In the middle of summer, when everybody's off work and knows that today is your rest day, it can be super difficult to pass up an invite like this, but just like with everything else, you can get better at saying no.

JOURNAL ENTRY—20:00

When it comes to your training, where do you feel the most peer pressure? Are you embarrassed to be the person asking the coach questions or to be the last one finishing a workout? Do your friends tell you to relax and have a beer and skip the Sunday morning workout? Would you like to start competing but don't think you're good enough?

The first time I got drunk, I was twelve years old, and a few of us were at my buddy's house after school. His parents had a closet full of room-temperature vodka from Costco, which we each used to fill our own Solo cups to the top. Then we pinched our noses, chugged it down, and waited to feel something. Before I did, though, the house phone rang. It was my dad. *Shouldn't you be getting ready for football practice?* he said. *No, that's Monday, Wednesday, Friday*, I said. *Yeah*, he said. *It's Wednesday.*

I sprinted home, threw my equipment into a bag, and hoped that my pads smelled enough to cover the alcohol on my breath. We were late, thankfully, so I ran to my dad's truck and rolled down the windows. I was already starting to sway, so I rested my head on the open window, and by the time we got there, I was so drunk I was stumbling across the field to catch up with the rest of the team.

I told my buddy what was happening, and he hooked his hand under my arm as we ran the warm-up lap. From there, word traveled fast, and when I'd go to line up in my three-point stance, the other guys would tap me from behind and watch me face-plant onto the field. From then on, if my buddies and I had a free period during school, even if it was at 9 a.m., we'd go back to that house and drink.

By high school, we were so well known for partying that a guidance counselor told us that we needed to slow down or someone was going to die. That didn't happen (at least not before we graduated), but there were plenty of DUIs, drunk-driving accidents, and kids messing around with oxy and heroin. I was never interested in hard drugs, and because I competed in a sport regulated by the US Anti-Doping Agency, which urine-tests all its athletes, I didn't smoke weed, either. But I had no problem drinking beer until I blacked out.

I'd never felt like I really fit in before, and I'm not sure if drinking convinced me that I did, or if I just stopped caring when I was drunk. Either way, it gave me the courage to talk to other kids at the party and have fun. And I had a lot of fun.

The third time I got a citation for drinking, my buddies and I were halfway to the state fair when we made a pit stop in a park to finish the case of beers in my backpack. When the cop shined his flashlight on us, we were so clearly busted that it wasn't even worth trying to run, but after he wrote us up, I did ask if we could keep the beer. He said no.

When I walked into the house that night, my dad was talking on the phone. I held up the citation and tried to explain what happened, but he waved me away. He wasn't angry. He wasn't surprised. He was disappointed in his own silent way, and that killed me.

I decided to get a handle on my drinking before I did something really stupid. And once I hit that switch, it was off entirely. In this case, it meant going cold turkey and cutting off all my old friends. I'd never been lonelier, but I eventually started going to AA meetings, which was a huge help. Vermont has one of the strongest sober communities in the country, and I met a group of guys I could go paintballing and dirt-biking with, so I didn't feel like I was missing out.

But that wasn't the case when I got to the OTC in Colorado Springs. I went to a few meetings there but didn't connect with anyone, so I carried my sobriety by myself. It was hard. I was away from my friends and family, the youngest guy on the team, and on the verge of getting kicked out if I didn't raise my numbers. Plus, my teammates weren't exactly understanding. *What do you mean, you won't have a beer with us?* they'd say while we all ate in the cafeteria. *Like, if I hit a new PR, you're not gonna celebrate with me?*

At first, I reacted by disengaging with them completely, but gradually I learned how to brush off their comments and even how to go out to the bars and not feel pressured to drink. I didn't make a big deal about it. I didn't try to convince anyone of anything. I just made it known that my decision wasn't up for discussion, which is a skill I've come back to throughout my CrossFit career.

Eating for Recovery

Even though Sammy took care of all the cooking when I was in-season, one of the most stressful parts of training was the volume of food I had to consume. A nutritionist told me that I needed about 10,000 calories a day, which meant that anytime I wasn't training or sleeping, I was eating. I'd wake up around 8 a.m., and by 8:05 I'd be having oatmeal with fruit and yogurt. An hour later, it'd be eggs, bacon, more fruit, and a bagel with cream cheese. Then, until my next meal, around 2:30 p.m., I'd be slamming protein shakes to keep my blood sugar up. In fact, during a normal day of training, I'd be drinking 2,000 to 3,000 calories, likely more than you eat in total. Then I'd go home and eat lunch, which was basically a mini-dinner, train again, and have my biggest meal of the day.

Cream Cheese Swirl Pumpkin Muffins

$1^3/_4$ cups all-purpose flour

1 tablespoon pumpkin spice

1 teaspoon baking soda

$^1/_2$ teaspoon salt

1 mashed banana

1 (15-ounce) can pumpkin puree

$1^1/_4$ cups granulated sugar, divided

$^1/_2$ cup firmly packed brown sugar

2 large eggs plus 1 large egg yolk, divided

$^1/_2$ cup coconut oil

1 tablespoon plus 2 teaspoons vanilla extract, divided

8 ounces cream cheese, at room temperature

1. Preheat the oven to 375°F. Line a muffin tin with paper liners and set aside.
2. Mix the dry ingredients in a medium bowl (the flour, pumpkin spice, baking soda, and salt). In a separate large bowl, mash the banana and mix with the pumpkin puree. Add 1 cup of the sugar, the brown sugar, whole eggs, oil, and 1 tablespoon of the vanilla, using a hand mixer to combine.
3. Add the dry ingredients to the wet. Mix until just combined. Pour the batter into the prepared muffin tin. Set aside.
4. Using the hand mixer, in a separate small bowl combine the cream cheese, the remaining $^1/_4$ cup granulated sugar, the yolk, and the remaining 2 teaspoons vanilla. Mix until smooth. Transfer the cream cheese to a resealable bag. Cut off a tiny hole

in the corner of the bag and use to pipe a dollop of sweetened cream cheese into each muffin cup. With a toothpick, swirl the cream cheese into batter. Do not overmix.

5. Bake for 18 to 20 minutes.
6. Cool for 5 minutes in the muffin tin, then move to a wire rack to finish cooling. Enjoy.

But it wasn't just the volume of food that was difficult. It was also the consistency I had to maintain. When I was first training, I'd skip breakfast, get dizzy during my afternoon session of lifting, then binge so hard that I'd have to wait an hour before I could get moving again. Needless to say, your body hates that kind of unpredictability, so I created a schedule for eating just like I developed a pattern for breathing. If your brain knows when it's going to get oxygen again, it relaxes, and you actually end up needing less oxygen. And if your body knows when you'll feed it again, it doesn't take every calorie it gets and store it as fat, which allows you to be a more efficient machine.

Blackberry Cheesecake Oat Bars

1½ cups blackberries

1 teaspoon lemon juice

½ cup plus 2 tablespoons granulated sugar, divided

¾ cup melted coconut oil

¾ cup light brown sugar

2 eggs, divided

3 teaspoons vanilla extract, divided

4 cups quick-cook oats

2 teaspoons cinnamon

2 teaspoons cornstarch

1 teaspoon baking soda

6 ounces cream cheese

¼ cup plain Greek yogurt

Pinch of salt

1. Preheat the oven to 350°F. Line a square 8-by-8-inch dish with parchment paper and set aside.
2. In a small bowl, toss the blackberries with the lemon juice and 2 tablespoons of the granulated sugar. Set aside while you prepare the remaining ingredients.
3. In a large bowl, beat the coconut oil, brown sugar, and ¼ cup of the granulated sugar using a hand mixer for 1 to 2 minutes. Add one egg and 2 teaspoons of the vanilla and beat until combined. Add the oats, cinnamon, cornstarch, and baking soda. Mix until well combined. Add all but 1 cup of the oat mixture to the square baking dish. Spread evenly throughout the dish and press firmly to create a crust.

4. In a separate medium bowl, beat the cream cheese, yogurt, and the remaining $1/4$ cup granulated sugar together for 1 to 2 minutes. Add the remaining egg and 1 teaspoon vanilla. Beat until combined. Pour the cheesecake layer over the oats and spread to evenly coat the crust.

5. Add the berries to the top of the cheesecake layer. Lastly, top with the remaining oats to create a crumble layer.

6. Bake for 35 to 40 minutes. Remove from the oven and allow to cool for 1 hour on the counter before slicing to serve.

If you want to consistently eat this volume of food, you can't wait until you're hungry. You have to approach your meals with the same determined mindset with which you approach your workouts, which often means ignoring the "I'm full" signals that are ricocheting through your brain. That's a risky road to walk down, because recognizing and listening to your body is a crucial part of being an athlete. So whether you're looking to lose weight or gain mass, I don't recommend that you go on an extreme diet, and unless you're an elite athlete competing at the highest levels, don't train yourself to eat whether you're hungry or not.

Strawberries in the Snow

16 ounces strawberries, thinly sliced

1 tablespoon granulated sugar

8 ounces cream cheese, at room temperature

8 ounces Cool Whip, thawed

1 cup powdered sugar

1 angel food cake, torn into bits

1. In a medium bowl, toss the sliced strawberries with the granulated sugar. Place the strawberries in the fridge for one hour.
2. In the bowl of a stand mixer add the cream cheese and Cool Whip. Beat for 2 minutes until combined and fluffy.
3. Slowly incorporate the powdered sugar and beat for an additional minute.
4. Either use mason jars or a trifle dish to layer: cake, Cool Whip, strawberry, REPEAT. Serve.

Games athletes can't eat just broccoli, brown rice, and chicken breast. To get 10,000 calories a day, you sometimes need to incorporate "unhealthy" foods, too, especially during competition. While others might weigh and measure every grain of brown rice after each event, I'd be eating a Snickers or mixing a gallon's worth of Gatorade powder into eight ounces of water—anything to re-up my blood sugar levels.

During training, Sammy always had an emergency stash of cookies in the freezer. And these were real cookies, not "healthy" cookies that used one cup of butter instead of two or covered everything in flaxseeds. When it was time for a treat at the end of the day, my philosophy was this: Cookies should have all the fat and sugar and calories they deserve. That way, when I eat them, I fully enjoy them and don't have to trick myself into thinking they're somehow healthy. And then during the off-season, I could really go to town.

Brown Butter Black Walnut Cinnamon Rolls

Dough

$^{1}/_{4}$ cup unsalted butter, browned

$^{3}/_{4}$ cup warm milk

$2^{1}/_{4}$ teaspoons quick-rise or active yeast

$^{1}/_{4}$ cup granulated sugar

1 egg plus 1 egg yolk, at room temperature

3 cups bread flour, plus more for dusting

$^{3}/_{4}$ teaspoon salt

$^{1}/_{2}$ teaspoon cinnamon

1 tablespoon olive oil

Filling

6 tablespoons salted butter at room temperature

$^{1}/_{2}$ cup brown sugar

2 teaspoons ground cinnamon

$^{1}/_{3}$ cup black walnuts, finely chopped

Cream Cheese Frosting

4 tablespoons salted butter, browned and cooled

4 ounces cream cheese, at room temperature

1 cup powdered sugar

1 teaspoon vanilla extract

$^{1}/_{4}$ teaspoon cinnamon

Pinch of kosher salt

1 to 2 tablespoons heavy cream or whole milk (optional)

1 teaspoon to 1 tablespoon flour (optional)

1. First, make the dough. Brown the butter in a skillet over medium heat until frothy and fragrant. Set aside to cool for 5 to 10 minutes.

2. In the bowl, of a stand mixer bowl, combine the warm milk, yeast, sugar, egg, egg yolk, and the slightly cooled browned butter. Mix for 30 seconds.

3. Add the bread flour, salt, and cinnamon. Knead for 5 minutes until the dough pulls away from the sides of the bowl.

4. Remove the dough from the bowl, drizzle the bowl with olive oil, and coat the sides. Return the dough to the bowl. Cover the bowl with plastic wrap or a damp kitchen towel and let rise for 1 to 2 hours, or until the dough has doubled in size.

5. Turn the dough out onto a lightly floured surface. Roll the dough out into a large rectangle until the dough is about $1/4$ inch thick. Wash and dry the mixer bowl and attachment.

6. Next, make the filling. Slather the dough with the softened butter. In a small bowl, mix the brown sugar and cinnamon. Evenly sprinkle the buttered surface with the brown sugar mixture. Last, sprinkle the chopped black walnuts.

7. Starting with the long edge farthest from you, roll the dough toward you, moving your fingers evenly back and forth along the dough, until it is rolled tightly, seam-side down. Cut into 9 to 12 rolls.

8. Place the rolls into a deep baking dish or cast-iron skillet. Loosely cover with plastic wrap and rest for 1 hour until puffed and risen (you could also proof

the dough in the fridge overnight for an amazing development of flavor and fluffy texture).

9. Preheat the oven to 375°F.

10. Bake for 20 to 22 minutes, until golden brown.

11. While the rolls are baking, make the cream cheese frosting. Brown the butter in a skillet over medium heat until frothy and fragrant. Set aside to cool for 5 to 10 minutes.

12. In the bowl of the stand mixer, beat the softened cream cheese for 30 seconds. Pour the cooled brown butter into the bowl along with the powdered sugar, vanilla, cinnamon, and salt. Beat for an additional 30 to 60 seconds until smooth. Add 1 to 2 tablespoons of heavy cream and 1 teaspoon to 1 tablespoon of flour, if needed, to achieve your desired consistency.

13. When the rolls have finished baking, remove them from the oven and allow to cool for 5 minutes before adding the frosting. Frost the rolls with the brown butter cream cheese frosting and serve.

Sometimes in the weeks after the Games, I'd eat an entire apple pie for breakfast. I wouldn't feel great afterward, but that wasn't the point. In fact, there were some foods that I looked forward to bingeing all season—like beef stroganoff made from the box—but most of the time, I wasn't eating for taste. Instead, I just wanted the freedom to eat whatever I wanted, whenever I wanted it. Sometimes that meant a family-sized baked good for breakfast and then nothing else until dinner. By the end of my off-season, I'd be so sick of desserts that I'd be ready to go back to spinach, rice, and grilled chicken again.

Skillet Apple Pie

2 Granny Smith apples, peeled and sliced

3 Honeycrisp apples, peeled and sliced

1 teaspoon lemon juice

2 teaspoons vanilla

$^1/_2$ cup granulated sugar

$^1/_4$ cup plus 1 tablespoon brown sugar, divided

1 teaspoon cinnamon

2 sheets store-bought pie crust

2 tablespoons salted butter, cubed

1 egg, beaten

Vanilla ice cream for serving (optional)

1. In a large bowl, toss the sliced apples with the lemon juice, vanilla, granulated sugar, $^1/_4$ cup of the brown sugar, and the cinnamon. Cover and rest in the fridge for 2 to 3 hours.
2. When ready to bake, preheat the oven to 350°F.
3. Lay one sheet of crust along the bottom of a seasoned cast-iron skillet. Pour the bowl of macerated apples onto the base of the pie. Add the cubes of butter along the top of the apples.
4. Top the pie with the second sheet of crust. Make it fancy with strips of crust or leave it whole, but be sure to cut vents in the crust to allow the steam to escape. Trim or tuck the edges of the crust.
5. Brush the top of the crust with the beaten egg and sprinkle with the remaining 1 tablespoon brown sugar.
6. Bake for 60 to 70 minutes until golden. Allow the pie to rest for 10 minutes before slicing and serving. Serve with a scoop of vanilla ice cream, if desired!

Emotional Recovery

The most important recovery I ever made was getting over the disappointment of 2015, and it was partly thanks to two things.

The big one was that I got to really hang out with Sammy for the first time the night that the Games ended. She and I had met a few years earlier when I visited the Reebok headquarters in Boston. That was where she worked, and I was so obviously into her that her co-worker gave me her number. But I didn't do anything with it because I was too chicken, so thankfully she reached out to me. We texted and called each other for a few months, but I was always so afraid that I was way more into her than she was into me that I eventually let the conversation fizzle out.

So when I saw her at the athlete check-in for the 2015 Games, I was rattled all over again, especially when she gave me a hug and held me a little longer than necessary. I texted her throughout the competition, which definitely didn't help me focus but did give me an idea on that Sunday, while I was moping around in the tunnel below the stadium at the end of the Games, wondering how I'd messed up so badly and taken silver for the second year in a row.

In that moment, I decided to go to the after-party that night to try to run into her. I usually hate crowds, and this was so out of character for me that when I told O'Keefe, he texted my friends to ask if I was all right.

I think O'Keefe figured it out pretty quickly when we walked into the party and I beelined straight for Sammy. She had to work that night, but afterward we went back to her hotel room and talked until I had to meet my family for brunch. On the way out of her room, I was so happy that I had to do everything I could not to say *I love you*, but thankfully she felt the same way, and we've been together ever since.

The next time you feel like you're at your lowest, you probably won't meet your life partner, but you may be able to do the other thing that helped me recover from the 2015 loss: a road trip.

After brunch with my family that Monday morning, I met up with two friends and Dan Bailey, another Games competitor, and we rented motorcycles from a nearby shop. Then we picked up food, tents, and sleeping bags and started riding with no destination in mind. Half the fun was not being prepared for whatever happened, whether it was getting caught in the rain or having to sleep in a parking lot because all the campsites had been booked months earlier.

After four days of the most intense exercising of your life, it may seem like the last thing you'd want to do is sit on a motorcycle in the rain. But it felt amazing not to have a plan—no workouts, no premade meals, no bedtime—and just to drive. There were no winners, no losers, no responsibilities, and no pressure to perform well. At the end of the day, I had a cellphone and a pocket of money, so the worst-case scenario was that we'd ride our motorcycles back to the shop and cut off the trip early.

All of that helped me unwind from the Games, and Dan Bailey gave me some perspective on the situation, too. At a diner, I remember him asking what I was so disappointed about. In two years, I'd gotten on the podium not just once, but twice, doing something that most competitive CrossFit athletes would work their whole lifetime to achieve but potentially never would. Though I understood what he was trying to do, I wasn't ready to hear it—at least not at that time. I'd wanted to win.

But over the course of my career, I've realized that disappointment is an unavoidable part of competing. If I'd made it to the Games in 2013, I probably would've quit as soon as we had to sit on the rower for an hour and a half. If I hadn't gotten pummeled by the ocean three years in a row, I would never have practiced my swimming. If I hadn't been embarrassed by the L-1 coach, I wouldn't have learned that the only clout you have in this sport is your ability to win. And if I hadn't blown a 100-plus-point lead in 2015, I would never have learned how to recover, and I wouldn't be the five-time CrossFit champion I am today.

And that's what made my decision to retire after the 2020 season an easy one. After five back-to-back victories, more than anyone else in the sport, I felt like I'd finally avenged that idiotic mistake from 2015. Over the seven years I competed in CrossFit, I won 29 events, 13 more than the guy after me, and earned 83 percent of all the possible points. In a sport where consistency matters above all else, my average placement during my entire career was 5.7, and during the five years that I won the Games, I finished 20th or worse only three times out of 73 total events.

I was undeniably the best, but even more important, I hadn't grown to hate the sport. That was what happened with weightlifting. Especially during the last year, I was so focused on proving everyone wrong and showing that I could recover from my back injury that I was running mostly on spite. I don't think I noticed how bad it had gotten until my last major meet, when I hit a 300-kilogram total. That's a huge milestone and one that I'd been chasing for most of my life, but I didn't feel ecstatic, accomplished, or relieved. I didn't really feel anything at all.

I never wanted to get to that point with CrossFit, and I also didn't want to exit the sport with a limp. Even though I'd recovered completely from fracturing both sides of my L-5, there was always a tiny part of me that worried about it cracking again, let alone the other 100 potential injuries that can come from moving massive amounts of weight as quickly as possible until you're on the verge of passing out.

So on one hand, it was difficult to leave. CrossFit is how I met my best friends, business partners, and even my wife. CrossFit was how I found the artist who tattooed my chest, how I was able to travel across the world, and how I bought the home we now live in.

Ever since the end of the 2015 season, CrossFit had been my world. And for that same reason, I was ready to leave. Except for those few weeks in August when I allowed myself a break, my focus was relentless. I'd passed up vacations, bachelor parties, and more dates with Sammy than I could count, all so I wouldn't miss a single training session or a full night of sleep.

For eight years, every day was roughly the same: wake up earlier than I'd like, sell my soul to the Assault Bike and the swimming intervals and the 40-minute AMRAPs, eat, sleep, repeat.

The hard work paid off. But I was ready to make decisions based on how they affected my family, friends, health, and happiness, not only my performance. After the 2020 Games, I had the most titles in history, my health, and seven years' worth of memories untainted by competing for the wrong reasons or desperately trying to hang on to my old glory. How many professional athletes can say the same?

ACKNOWLEDGMENTS

Thank you, Matt O'Keefe, for being by my side from day one. None of this would have been possible without you.

This has been my world and part of my life journey. I hope that you have enjoyed reading it and perhaps have had some insights along the way. Pursue your path and use *HWPO* as a guide. LFG.

ADDITIONAL MAT FRASER WORKOUTS

Strength

Snatches

Power Snatch
2 @ 80%
3 @ 85%
1 @ 90%
2 @ 85%
2 sets of 3 @ 80%

Snatch
4 sets
1 snatch + 1 hang snatch
Start @ 70–75%

Snatch
3 @ 80%
2 @ 85%
2 sets of 2 @ 80%

Snatch
3 sets of 5 @ 215 lbs
3 sets of 4 @ 225 lbs
3 sets of 3 @ 275 lbs

Snatch Balance
2 @ 80%
2 sets of 2 @ 85%
1 @ 90%
3 sets of 2 @ 75%

Cleans

3-Position Power Clean
6 sets (ground, below the knee, above the knee)
5 @ 65% (increase if safe)

Hang Power Clean
Every 2 mins for 6 sets
2 hang power cleans + 1 hang squat clean
Start @ 70% of power clean

Power Clean
3 @ 80%
2 sets of 3 @ 85%
4 sets of 3 @75%

Power Clean
3 sets of 3
(start heavy, add 10 lbs each set)

Press and Jerks

Strict Press
2 sets of 3 @ 80%
2 @ 85%
3 sets of 3 @ 80%

4 Sets Every 3 Mins
7 strict presses @ 65–75%
10 dual dumbbell push jerks (heavy)

Clean and Jerk
(2 cleans + 1 jerk)
@ 75%
@ 80%
@ 85%
@ 80%

Squats

Front Squat
5 @ 60%
5 @ 65%
2 sets of 5 @ 70%

Back Squat
8 @ 65%
8 @ 70%
8 @75%
8 @ 80%

Back Squat
8 @ 65%
8 @ 70%
6 @ 80%
6 @ 85%

Front Squat
5 @ 70%
5 @ 75%
5 @ 80%
5 @ 85%

Overhead Squat
Every 2 mins for 6 sets
3 @ 80%
2 sets of 3 @ 85%
3 sets of 4 @ 75%

Front Squat
5 @ 60%
5 @ 70%
5 @ 75%
5 @ 80%

Back Squat
8 @ 65%
8 @ 70%
6 @ 80%
6 @ 85%

Overhead Squat
Every 90 secs for 6 sets
Set 1: 5 reps @ 80%
Sets 2–4: 3 reps @ 85%
Sets 5–6: 4 reps @ 75%

Barbell Conditioning

EMOM for 8 Mins
3 power cleans (medium-light)
3 thrusters (medium)
3 power jerks (medium)

Accessories

Bench Press
5 sets of 3 dead stop
(start heavy, add 10 lbs each set)

5 Rounds
Dumbbell complex
5 power cleans (heavy)
4 front squats (heavy)
3 shoulder-to-overheads (heavy)
Rest: 2 mins between rounds

4 Sets
200 ft yoke
100 ft hand-over-hand sled pull
Rest: 90 secs

EMOM for 10 Mins
8 strict pull-ups with 10 lb vest

Endurance

BikeErg

4 Sets
8:00 255–272 watts
2:00 204–221 watts

Conditioning
20 mins alternating
Odd mins: 21 cal bike
Even mins: 6 deficit handstand
    push-ups
Complete bike in under 49 secs

Conditioning
2 rounds for time
50 toes-to-bars
40 thrusters (light)
40/30 cal rows

For time
150 double-unders
50 pull-ups

Grip work
Accumulate 4 mins top of
    deadlift (bar is 50% of body
    weight)

3 Sets
3,200 m 290 watts damper 6.5
    (bike erg)
Run 800 m

Every 8 mins for 4 sets
2,200m BikeErg
600m SkiErg

EMOM for 62 mins
Odd mins: 20 cal row
Even mins: 15 burpees

5 Sets
600m ski
400m run
30 push-ups
Rest: 1 min

For time
3,000m 30 lb Ruck
Rest: 2 mins
3,000m run
21 thrusters (medium)
21 burpee pull-ups
9 thrusters (heavy)
Rest: 2 mins
40 cal row
10 squat cleans (medium)
10 box step-overs
30 strict handstand push-ups

4 Sets
200 ft farmer's carry
800m run
3,000m row
800m run
3,000m row
800m run

Row

3 sets
750m 1:40
550m 1:38
350m 1:36
200m hard
Rest: 1 min between intervals
Rest: 3 mins between sets
Rest: 5 mins
Then
5 sets
250m hard
Rest: 30 secs

Every 7 mins for 4 sets

1,000m bike
30 strict handstand push-ups
1,000m bike
20 strict handstand push-ups

For time

75 cal row
60 wall-ball (M 30 lbs/W 20 lbs)
40 cal BikeErg
30 dumbbell thrusters (heavy)

Speed

8 sets
400m run sub 1:20
Rest: 1 min

6 sets (BikeErg)
8 cal seated damper 4
12 cal standing damper 10

10 sets
500m row
Rest: 1 min

5 sets
Big hill sprints
25 air squats

:30 On/:30 Off
20 rounds for max cal on Assault
    Bike
13 rounds @ 600 watts
7 rounds @ 700 watts

3 sets
1,100m row
Rest: 2:00

4 sets
550m row
Rest: 1:00

EMOM for 12 mins
Odd mins: 15 cal bike standing
Even mins: 15 burpees

3 sets
:75 on/1:45 off
20/15 Echo Bike
Max parallette facing burpees

Row
6 sets for max cal
3:00 on/2:00 off

3 sets, Assault Bike
:30 340 watts
:30 easy
Rest
5 sets
:30 510 watts damper 10
4:30 312 watts
2:00 easy

Every 4 mins for 4 sets
Assault Bike
25 cal

C2 Bike

3 sets

:30 damper 0
:30 damper 5
:30 damper 10 stand

3 sets

3 mins 357 watts 105 rpm
2 mins easy

Rest 2 mins

2 mins 374 watts damper (5–6)
    110 rpm
2 mins easy
3 mins 357 watts damper (7–8)
    105 rpm
2 mins easy
4 mins 357 watts damper (10)
    105 rpm
2 mins easy
3 mins 357 damper (7–8)
    105 rpm
2 mins easy
2 mins 374 damper (5–6)
5 min 290 watts

4 min 323 watts
3 min 340 watts
Rest: 3:00
4 min 306 watts
3 min 323 watts
2 min 340 watts
Rest: 3:00
3 min 340 watts
2 min 367 watts
1 min 375 watts
Rest: 3:00

3 sets

1 min 400 watts damper 10
Rest: 1:00

Coordination

EMOM for 10 mins
Odd mins: Handstand walk
  obstacles up and back
Even mins:
10 dumbbell bench presses
  (M 85 lbs/W 55 lbs)

Ring Muscle-Up with Vest
7–5–3–5–7 unbroken 1st one
  strict

Every 4 Mins for 4–6 Sets
4/3 pegboard
6L/6R dumbbell push presses
  (heavy)

7 Rounds
5 hang power snatches
  (medium)
5 overhead squats (medium)
5 bar muscle-ups

8 Sets
20 ft legless rope climb with vest

EMOM for 21 mins
Minute 1: 21 cal run
Minute 2: 16 toes-to-bars
Minute 3: 50 ft handstand
  (walk up and back obstacles)

For time
40 strict handstand push-ups
60 GHD
80 wall-balls
100 heavy double-unders

EMOM for 10 mins
3 strict muscle-ups

Strict Muscle-Up with Vest
5 × 5

5 Rounds
30 heavy double-unders
10 bar-facing burpees
5 power snatches
  (medium-heavy)

HWPO WORKOUT LOG

Below are some of the most popular benchmark workouts in CrossFit. They're meant to be tested every few months in order to track your progress and identify your weaknesses. As always, you should scale the movements and weight as needed.

When there are weights included, the first number is considered the Rx weight for men, and the second number is the Rx weight for women.

Workout	Date	Score	Weight	Notes
ANGIE For Time 100 Pull-Ups, 100 Push-Ups, 100 Sit-Ups, 100 Air Squats				
ANNIE For Time 50–40–30–20–10 Reps Double-Unders and Sit-Ups				
BARBARA For Time 5 Rounds Rest: 3 Minutes Between Rounds 20 Pull-Ups, 30 Push-Ups, 40 Sit-Ups, 50 Air Squats				

Workout	Date	Score	Weight	Notes
CHELSEA EMOM for 30 Minutes 5 Pull-Ups, 10 Push-Ups, 15 Air Squats				
CINDY AMRAP in 20 Minutes 5 Pull-Ups, 10 Push-Ups, 15 Air Squats				
DIANE For Time 21–15–9 Reps Deadlifts (M 225 lbs/W155 lbs) and Handstand Push-Ups				
ELIZABETH For Time 21–15–9 Reps Cleans (M 135 lbs /W 95 lbs) and Ring Dips				
EVA For Time 5 Rounds 800m Run, 30 Kettlebell Swings (M 32 kg/W 24 kg), 30 Pull-Ups				
FRAN For Time 21–15–9 Reps Thrusters (M 95 lbs /W 65 lbs) and Pull-Ups				
GRACE For Time 30 Reps Clean and Jerks (M 135 lbs/W 95 lbs)				

Workout	Date	Score	Weight	Notes
HELEN For Time 3 Rounds 400m Run, 21 Kettlebell Swings (M 24 kg/W 16 kg), 12 Pull-Ups				
ISABEL For Time 30 Snatches (M 135 lbs/W 95 lbs)				
JACKIE For Time 1,000m Row, 50 Thrusters (M 45 lbs /W 35 lbs), 30 Pull-Ups				
KAREN For Time 150 Walls-Balls (M 20 lbs/W 14 lbs)				
KELLY For Time 5 Rounds 400m Run, 30 Box Jumps (M 24″/W 20″), 30 Wall-Balls (M 20 lbs /W 14 lbs)				
LINDA For Time 10—9—8—7—6—5—4—3—2—1 Reps 1½ × Bodyweight Deadlift, Bodyweight Bench Press, ¾ × Bodyweight Cleans				
LYNNE AMRAP for 5 Rounds Max Bodyweight Bench Press and Max Pull-Ups				

Workout	Date	Score	Weight	Notes
MARY AMRAP in 20 Minutes 5 Handstand Push-Ups, 10 Pistols (Alternating Legs), 15 Pull-Ups				
NANCY For Time 5 Rounds 400m Run and 15 Overhead Squats (M 95 lbs/W 65 lbs)				
NICOLE AMRAP in 20 Minutes 400m Run and Max Pull-Ups (Score is total pulls-ups completed in all rounds)				

GLOSSARY

1RM—one-rep max; the heaviest you've every lifted in a certain movement

AMRAP—as many reps as possible; a workout type that's always paired with a time domain (15 minutes, AMRAP)

Burpee—a conditioning exercise in which a person squats, places the palms of the hands on the floor in front of the feet, jumps back into a push-up position, in some cases completes one push-up, returns to the squat position, then jumps up into the air while extending the arms overhead

Butterfly—a style of doing pull-ups and chest-to-bars where you link reps by swinging in a circular motion

Chest-to-Bar—a pull-up, but your collarbone (or lower on your chest) has to touch the bar. Can be done strict, kipping, or butterfly

Chipper—a workout with a number of different movements, typically between 5 and 10, performed at high volume, one after the other, until the workout is completed

EMOM—every minute on the minute; a workout type that prescribes a workload that has to be completed within the minute, and the rest of the time is for rest. Variations include E2MOM (every two minutes on the minute), E3MOM, etc.

FTP—functional threshold power: the highest effort you can sustain for one hour, measured as watts on a stationary bike

GHD—a machine specifically designed for you to do sit-ups with a larger range of motion

Jerk vs. Push—jerk means you bend your legs and drop underneath the bar during the movement, whereas push means you do not

Kipping—a movement done with the help of a swing or a hip thrust

METCON—metabolic conditioning

OHS—overhead squat

Pistols—a one-legged air squat

Power vs. Squat—power means you don't squat below parallel during the movement (e.g., a power snatch), whereas squat means you do

PR—your "personal record," the fastest time you've completed a workout, the most reps you've ever done of an exercise, or the same thing as a 1RM if you're talking about a lift

Regionals—the second phase of the CrossFit season, typically in person and divided into regions

Rx—as the workout is written, including the weight and the number of reps

Scaled—a modified version of the workout, including less weight or fewer reps

STOH—shoulder to overhead; a broad term that allows you to choose your preferred way to get a weight from your shoulders to over your head, whether that means a strict press, push press, or jerk

Strict—a movement done using only the necessary muscles and with no extra help from your hips or a swing

The Games—the sport's annual competition and traditionally for only the most elite forty or so athletes

The Open—the CrossFit Open, a worldwide, multiweek, remote competition that's the first phase of the CrossFit season

Thruster—a front squat with a push press at the top

Toes-to-Bar—a movement where you hang from a bar and bring your feet to the bar. Can be performed strict or kipping